ECG CASE STUDIES

Second

D1239386

100 CHALLENGING
ELECTROCARDIOGRAMS

BY

JULIAN FRIEDEN, M.D., F.A.C.P., F.A.C.C.
Attending Physician, Department of Medicine
Cardiology Service
Physician-in-Charge, Coronary Care Unit
Montefiore Hospital and Medical Center
Associate Clinical Professor of Medicine
Albert Einstein College of Medicine
New York, New York

AND

IRA L. RUBIN, M.D., F.A.C.P., F.A.C.C.
Attending Physician, Department of Medicine
Cardiology Service
Head, ECG Department
Montefiore Hospital and Medical Center
Clinical Professor of Medicine
Albert Einstein College of Medicine
New York, New York

 Medical Examination Publishing Co., Inc.
an Excerpta Medica company

969 Stewart Avenue • Garden City, New York 11530

Library of Congress
Catalog Card Number
77-94387

ISBN 0-87488-003-3

October, 1974

PRINTED IN THE UNITED STATES OF AMERICA

ECG CASE STUDIES
Second Edition

TABLE OF CONTENTS

PREFACE TO THE FIRST EDITION

The electrocardiogram is a simple and convenient technique for the detection of cardiac problems. To treat cardiac patients efficiently, an accurate interpretation is essential. Prompt evaluation of the electrocardiogram is often necessary, especially to fully utilize the advantages of intensive care units.

This book is intended to help the physician in reviewing and broadening his knowledge of electrocardiography. It is not a textbook, as many excellent texts are available. The cases presented cover a wide range of commonly encountered problems. They are designed to develop the physician's ability to analyze an electrocardiogram with a brief clinical history as background.

The book consists of 100 questions and answers: both arrhythmias and contour changes are presented. The answers will aid the reader in correlating the clinical and electrocardiographic data. In the complicated cases, a detailed analysis of the electrocardiogram is given.

PREFACE TO THE SECOND EDITION

Since publication of the first edition of ECG Case Studies in 1969, clinical electrocardiography remains the most important noninvasive technique in clinical cardiology. Refinements in the field have improved understanding of the electrocardiogram as an indicator of the pathophysiology of the heart. This knowledge has been particularly helpful in understanding arrhythmias, hemiblocks, heart block and pacemakers. We have attempted to include electrocardiograms illustrating many of these points, as well as the more commonly occurring electrocardiographic patterns and rhythms. None of the electrocardiograms in this edition were published in the previous edition.

Many of these cases have been published in the *New York State Journal of Medicine* and some will be published in the future. We wish to thank Dr. Alfred A. Angrist, Editor of the *New York State Journal of Medicine,* for his courtesy in allowing us to use this material.

We would like to express our appreciation to Mrs. Esther Rockett for her excellent secretarial assistance in the preparation of this book.

J. F.
I. L. R.

To our wives, Nancy and Beatrice

CASE STUDY 1: QUESTION

The patient was an asymptomatic sixty year-old man who had been told of electrocardio-graphic abnormalities following a routine examination. What is the interpretation?

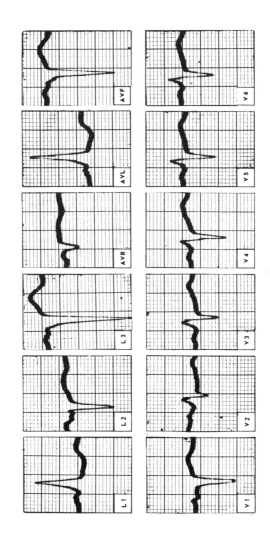

CASE STUDY 1: ANSWER

The rhythm is sinus rhythm. In leads I and aVl, the P-R interval is very short (0.10 second), and the QRS complex has a slurred initial component. The P-R interval in V_1 appears longer, since the initial portion of the QRS in this lead is isoelectric. The combination of a short P-R interval, QRS duration of 0.14 second, and initial slurring (Delta wave) of the QRS complex is characteristic of the Wolff-Parkinson-White syndrome. (Type B) Such patients, while often suffering from recurrent arrhythmias, may be completely asymptomatic.

CASE STUDY 2: QUESTION

What is the rhythm? (This tracing was obtained from a monitor in the CCU).

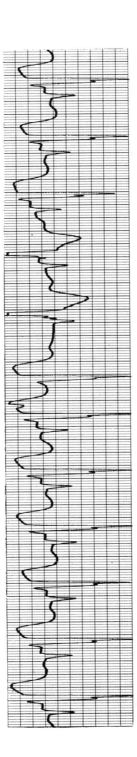

CASE STUDY 2: ANSWER

The rhythm is regular sinus for the first six beats. The giant P waves and high voltage QRS complex are due to distortion of the non-standardized monitor lead. The sixth QRS is followed by a premature ectopic atrial beat with prolongation of the P-R and slightly aberrant conduction of the initial .02 second of the following QRS. The ensuing beat is a ventricular escape beat occurring immediately following the sinus P wave and is obviously not conducted from this. The next QRS is also a ventricular escape preceded by a non-conducted P wave. Sinus rhythm then resumes. The diagnosis is sinus rhythm with a premature atrial contraction (with prolongation of the P-R and slightly aberrant intra-ventricular conduction). In addition, there are ventricular escape beats followed by re-sumption of sinus rhythm.

CASE STUDY 3: QUESTION

What is the interpretation of this electrocardiogram? The patient was a fifty-six-year-old man admitted to the hospital with recurrent chest pain. The present electrocardiogram is unchanged from a tracing taken one month before.

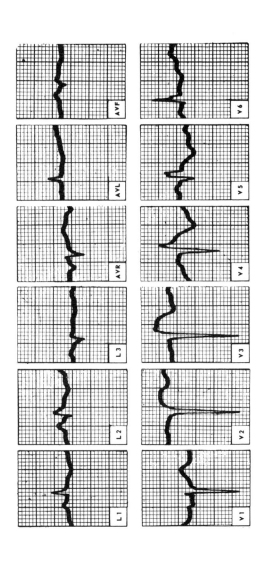

The rhythm is regular sinus rhythm with S-T elevations in leads I, II, III, aVf, and V₂ to V₆. T is inverted in these leads. There is an abnormal Q wave in leads II, III, aVf, V₅, and V₆. In leads V₂ to V₄ there is a QS pattern. The S-T segment is bowed upward and elevated in leads I, II, V₂ to V₅. These abnormalities are secondary to multiple infarctions. Since the tracing is unchanged from previous records, recent infarction cannot be diagnosed from the electrocardiogram. Patients with persistent patterns of abnormal Q waves with elevated S-T segments often have a ventricular aneurysm.

CASE STUDY 4: QUESTION

What is the rhythm? The patient has not been receiving any cardiac drugs. The electrocardiogram was obtained during the course of monitoring this patient with an acute myocardial infarction.

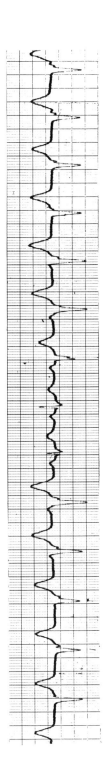

CASE STUDY 4: ANSWER

P waves are visible preceding QRS complexes #6, 7, and 8. The P wave is not so clear-ly seen, but is visible preceding beats #5 and 9 and then becomes buried in the other QRS complexes. The initial 5 QRS complexes are wide and aberrant, but are not at a rapid rate (80 per minute). These idioventricular beats are termed accelerated idioventricu-lar rhythm. The rhythm has been called isorhythmic dissociation; it is usually benign and does not require therapy. Beat #8 is preceded by a P wave with a short P-R inter-val and has a configuration different from both beats 7 and 9. It is a fusion beat, con-firming the presence of a parasystolic focus.

CASE STUDY 5: QUESTION

What is the rhythm? Lead 3.

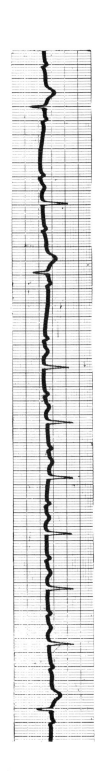

CASE STUDY 5: ANSWER

The P-P intervals are regular at a rate of 80 per minute. The P-R intervals of beats #2-7 and beat #9 are prolonged to .38 sec. The P waves following QRS #7 and 9 are non-conducted. Following these non-conducted P waves, the P-R shortens to .21 second and the succeeding QRS is aberrant. The shortened P-R interval is due to the prolonged pause following the blocked P wave which allows recovery of AV conduction. The variation in QRS configuration is also probably related to the duration of the R-R interval. The rhythm is regular sinus rhythm, 1st and 2nd degree heart block.

CASE STUDY 6: QUESTION

What is the interpretation? These two electrocardiograms (lead 2) were obtained ten minutes apart in a patient with chest pain.

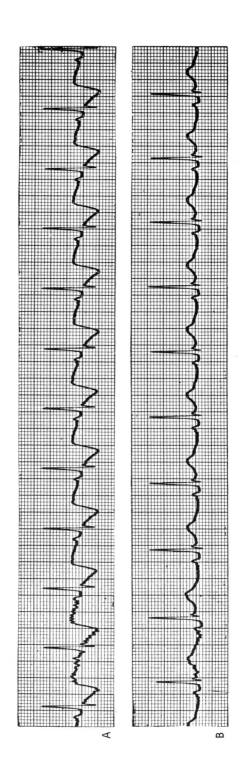

A

B

CASE STUDY 6: ANSWER

Strip 1 shows S-T depression with T inversion. The abnormalities indicate myocardial ischemia. The second tracing obtained when the pain has disappeared is a normal lead 2. Patients with angina often have S-T abnormalities occurring during their pain which are helpful diagnostically, as they may occur in a patient whose resting tracing is normal. Exercise may induce these changes when the resting electrocardiogram is normal.

CASE STUDY 7: QUESTION

What is the rhythm? The tracing was obtained while monitoring a patient with acute myocardial infarction in the Coronary Care Unit.

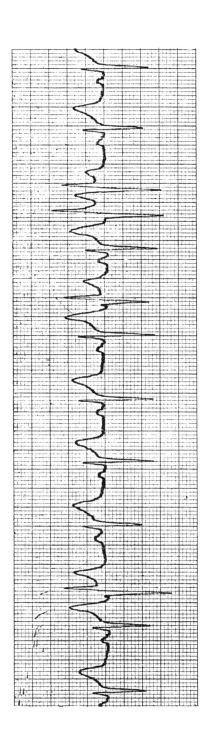

CASE STUDY 7: ANSWER

Beat #3 is premature and is preceded by a T wave which is deformed and more peaked than usual, due to a superimposed P wave. Note that this QRS complex is slightly aberrant. This is, therefore, an atrial premature contraction with aberrant ventricular conduction. Beat #8 is a similar premature beat and beats #10 and 11 are a pair of premature atrial contractions. The initial .04 sec. of premature beats #10 and 11 is negative and represents a Q wave. This may be evidence of myocardial infarction, or may simply represent aberrant ventricular conduction. Premature atrial beats are usually benign, but in this setting, may be a precursor to a supraventricular tachycardia or atrial fibrillation.

CASE STUDY 8: QUESTION

What is the diagnosis in this 82 year-old man who was admitted to the hospital having had a syncopal seizure?

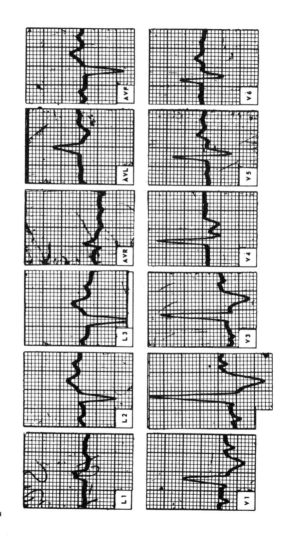

CASE STUDY 8: ANSWER

The rhythm is a regular sinus rhythm with a PR interval of .21 seconds. The QRS duration is .14 seconds. In the limb leads, the QRS configuration is that of left bundle branch block, but in the precordial leads, there is a tall R wave in V1 and a deep S wave in V6 consistent with right bundle branch block. This represents bilateral bundle branch block. It is often a precursor of transient or permanent complete heart block. With these findings in a symptomatic patient a permanent pacemaker is usually indicated. Anteroseptal infarction is often present, particularly when there are Q waves in V1 and V2, as in this case. However, in this patient, the Q waves are small and not diagnostic of infarction.

CASE STUDY 9: QUESTION

The patient is a 68 year-old man with a history of hypertension and a myocardial infarction four years prior to this record. What is the diagnosis?

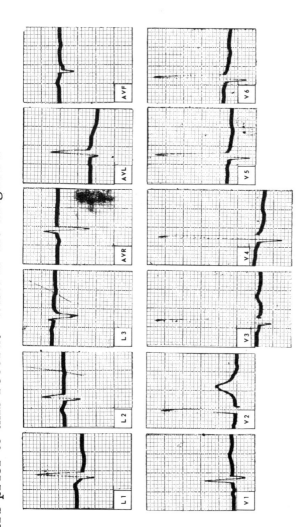

CASE STUDY 9: ANSWER

The rhythm is regular sinus rhythm. In leads 1, 2, AVL, and V_{3-6}, there is a narrow but rather deep Q wave. The S-T segment is depressed in lead 1 and slightly elevated in leads 2, 3, and V_{4-6} with T inverted. There is a dominant R wave in V_1 and high precordial voltage in the remaining precordial leads. There is counterclockwise rotation of the heart electrically. These findings are compatible with an old myocardial infarction, probably involving the anterolateral and possibly inferior wall. The tall R wave in V_1 suggests that the postero-lateral wall may be involved as well. The tracing demonstrates that narrow and deep Q waves may be significant even when their duration does not reach .04 sec. The high voltage suggests left ventricular hypertrophy.

CASE STUDY 10: QUESTION

The patient is a 42 year-old woman with a history of many years of anterior chest pain of a somewhat atypical nature. The patient's pain has been present and relatively stable for a number of years, and this electrocardiographic picture is a stable one. What is the diagnosis?

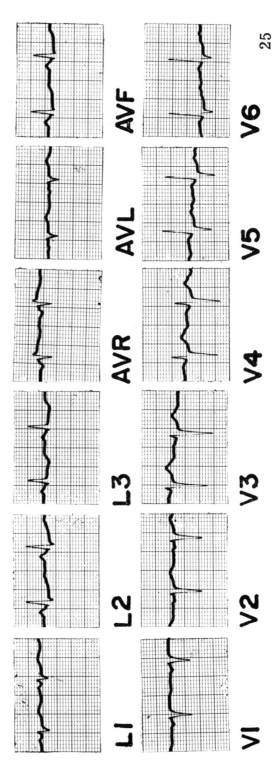

CASE STUDY 10: ANSWER

The rhythm is regular sinus rhythm. The mean electrical axis is $+90^\circ$. The ST is depressed in leads 2, 3, AVF, and V_{4-6}. These are non-specific abnormalities. A large group of relatively young women with non-specific ST abnormalities and atypical pain, has recently been studied with coronary angiograms. These patients, particularly if all risk factors are negative, commonly do not have significant coronary heart disease. The electrocardiographic findings in an apprehensive, anxious, relatively young woman, are usually not indicative of significant heart disease.

NOTES

CASE STUDY 11: QUESTION

What is the rhythm?

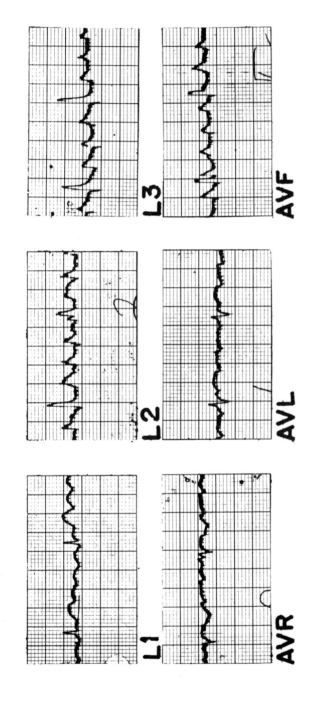

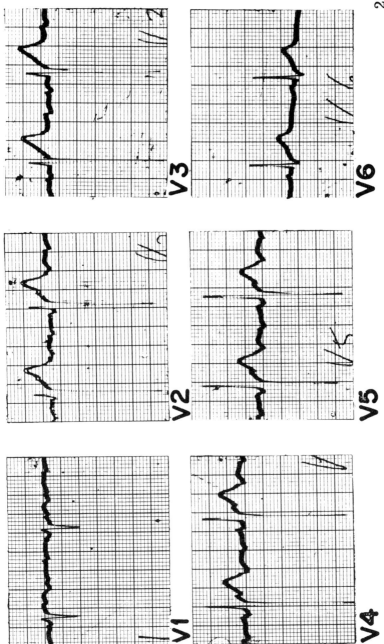

CASE STUDY 11: ANSWER

The ventricular rhythm is regular in all leads. In leads 2, 3 and AVF and less clearly in V4 and V5, regular recurring undulations of the baseline are seen. These occur at a regular rate of approximately 250 a minute. These undulations resemble atrial flutter. In V6 no undulations are seen, and P waves are clearly visible before each QRS; the ventricular rate has not changed. The undulations must be artifacts, since if the rhythm had gone from flutter to sinus rhythm the ventricular rate would have changed. This patient had a severe parkinsonian tremor.

CASE STUDY 12: QUESTION

The patient, a thirty-seven year-old woman, was admitted to the hospital with fever and vague chest pain. What is the interpretation?

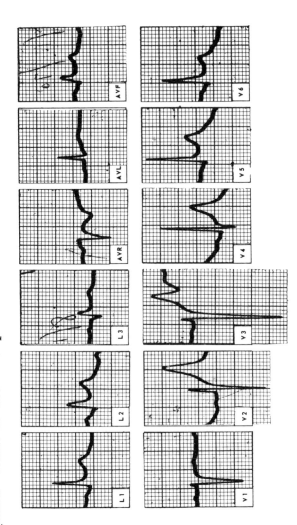

The rhythm is a regular sinus rhythm. In leads I, II, III, aVf, V$_5$, and V$_6$, S-T is elevated. These S-T elevations are suspicious of pericarditis, although they may occur early in the course of an acute myocardial infarct. Occasionally, in younger patients particularly, they may be seen as a normal variant. Serial observations demonstrated that this patient did indeed have a viral pericarditis. The T waves became inverted, and the S-T segments returned to the base line.

The first two beats are widely aberrant and preceded by a pacemaker spike. They are followed by two premature beats with a different QRS configuration which are ventricular extrasystoles. These extrasystoles suppress the pacemaker, which then begins beating following the second extrasystole. After two pacemaker beats, ventricular tachycardia ensues at an irregular rate of approximately 150 beats/min. This spontaneously disappears and a pacemaker rhythm with ventricular premature contractions then recurs. There are retrograde P waves on the ascending limbs of the T wave of these paced beats. In view of the ventricular irritability, the pacemaker rate should be accelerated and, in this way, often the extrasystoles can be suppressed and the ventricular tachycardia prevented. If this fails, antiarrhythmic drug therapy can be given. A pacemaker which is inhibited by early spontaneous ventricular activity is a demand pacemaker.

CASE STUDY 14: QUESTION

The patient is a 52 year-old man admitted to the hospital for elective surgery. What is the interpretation of this electrocardiogram?

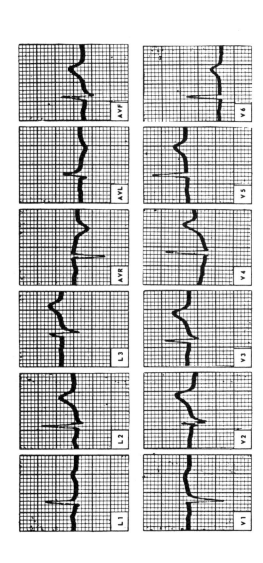

CASE STUDY 14: ANSWER

In the standard leads, T3 is taller than T1. In AVL, a small q is present with S-T slightly elevated and T inverted. In V2, a small q and splintered QRS is visible. These abnormalities suggest anterior infarction of indeterminate age. A T wave in lead 3 taller than lead 1 when the heart is horizontal, is an abnormal finding of a non-specific nature.

CASE STUDY 15: QUESTION

What is the interpretation of this arrhythmia? (lead 2)

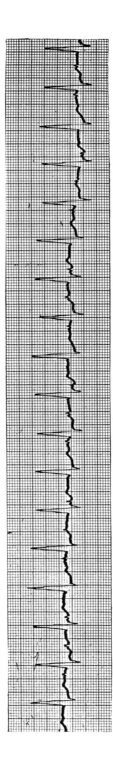

CASE STUDY 15: ANSWER

The ventricular rate is regular at 105 beats per minute. The atrial rate is also regular at 145 beats per minute and totally independent of the ventricular complexes. The rhythm, therefore, is a double tachycardia with the atrial rate faster than the ventricular rate. Since the QRS complexes are aberrant, and measure greater than .12 second, they must originate either below the bifurcation of the bundle of His, or if above the bifurcation, they are conducted with aberration.

Since the ventricular rate is only 105, this is probably not a true ventricular tachycardia, but could be categorized as a slow ventricular tachycardia or accelerated idioventricular rhythm.

CASE STUDY 16: QUESTION

What is the rhythm? Continuous lead 2.

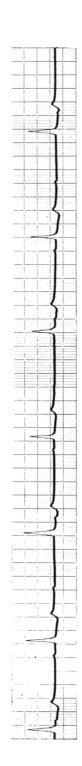

CASE STUDY 16: ANSWER

The P-P interval is perfectly regular. The R-R interval varies slightly. Each of the early QRS complexes (beats #2, 4 and 6) is preceded by a P wave with a fixed P-R interval of .20 sec. All other P waves are blocked and there are junctional escapes occurring at precisely regular R-R intervals. The rhythm is sinus rhythm with A-V dissociation and occasional capture. This electrocardiogram represents a high degree of A-V block (Mobitz II). Patients with this arrhythmia usually require a cardiac pacemaker.

CASE STUDY 17: QUESTION

What is the rhythm? (lead I)

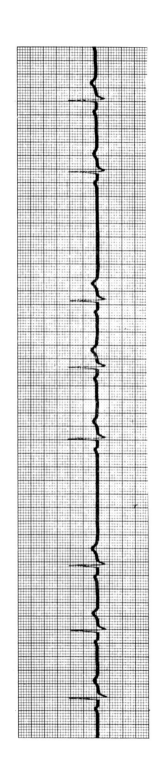

CASE STUDY 17: ANSWER

The first 3 beats are sinus beats at a rate of 65/min. Beat #4 is preceded by a long pause which is almost precisely double the usual P-P interval. It is preceded by a P wave of normal configuration. Following beat #6 the long pause recurs. The diagnosis is either sino-atrial block or sinus arrest. When the pause is exactly double the normal P-P interval, sino-atrial block is probable.

CASE STUDY 18: QUESTION

What is the interpretation? The patient is a 70 year-old man admitted with congestive heart failure.

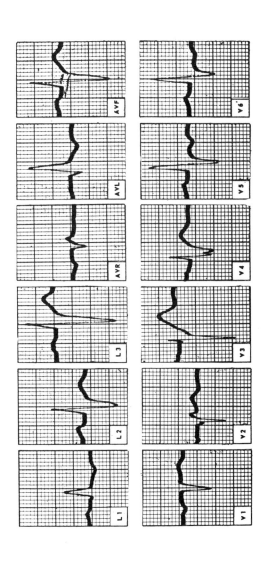

CASE STUDY 18: ANSWER

The rhythm is regular sinus rhythm with a P-R interval of .24 second. The QRS duration is .16 second. There is left axis deviation beyond -30°. A q is present in leads 1 and AVL with T inverted. In V_2, there is a deep Q wave with notching of the initial portion of the downstroke. There is a QS in V_1. T is inverted in V_5 and V_6. The patient has an intraventricular conduction defect which is not left bundle branch block, since there are Q waves in leads 1 and AVL. There is left axis deviation which implies left anterior hemiblock. The slurred Q in V_2 is highly suspicious of anteroseptal infarction. The diffuse S-T and T wave abnormalities indicate myocardial damage. The deep Q in AVL suggests lateral wall infarction. There is 1° A-V block.

CASE STUDY 19: QUESTION

The patient is a 60 year-old woman with a history of hypertension and long-standing renal disease. She has a history of a myocardial infarction 2 years ago. What is the interpretation of this electrocardiogram obtained on admission to the hospital?

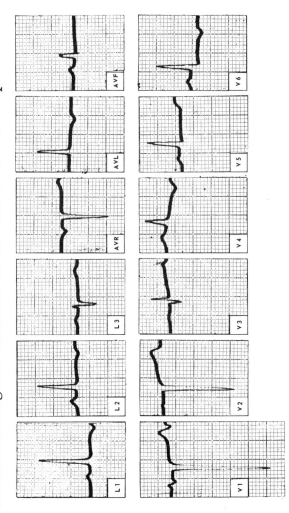

CASE STUDY 19: ANSWER

The rhythm is regular sinus rhythm. The S wave in V_1 is deep, measuring 27 mm. There is a QS in V_1 and V_2, and a deep Q wave in V_3. The T wave is inverted in leads 1, 2, AVL, and V_{4-6} with a prolonged ST segment, and a total Q-T duration of .46 sec.

The high voltage in V_1 is suggestive, but not diagnostic of left ventricular hypertrophy. The QS patterns in $V_{1\&2}$ with a deep Q in V_3 suggest anteroseptal infarction of indeterminate age. The prolonged Q-T segment with the rather narrow T wave, and a flat prolonged ST segment, is a finding often associated with hypocalcemia. The patient's calcium was 7.5 mgm%.

NOTES

CASE STUDY 20: QUESTION

Simultaneous V1, V2 and V3 – What is the rhythm?

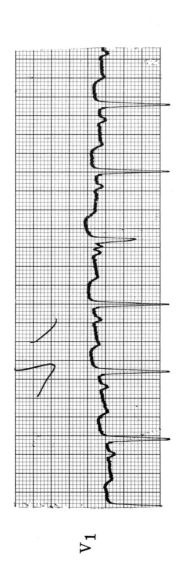

V1

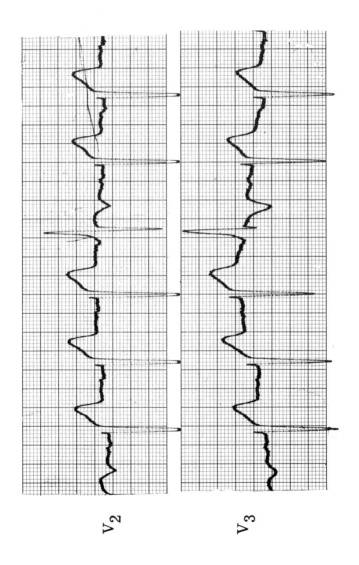

CASE STUDY 20: ANSWER

The 4th QRS complex is aberrant and appears premature. It is preceded by a P wave which is similar to the usual P wave and is precisely on time. In V_2 and V_3 the initial slurring of the QRS complexes in this beat resembles a delta wave. The slurring appears as a negative wave in V_1. This aberrantly conducted beat is either anomalous conduction of a sinus P wave of a Wolff-Parkinson-White variety, or a premature beat of the ventricle (or the A-V junction with aberrant ventricular conduction). In order to differentiate these two interpretations, monitoring would be necessary. If the aberrant beat arises in the ventricle, its relationship to the P wave will vary when the sinus rate changes.

CASE STUDY 21: QUESTION

The patient was a seventy year-old woman admitted to the hospital with severe weakness and long-standing congestive failure. She had received diuretic therapy and digitalis. What is the interpretation of this admission electrocardiogram? The ventricular rate was 70 per minute.

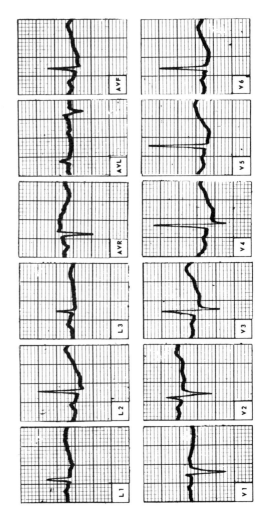

CASE STUDY 21: ANSWER

The tracing shows regular sinus rhythm. There is a striking abnormality in the precordial leads where large U waves are visible. The S-T segments are slightly depressed, and in V_3 to V_6 the T wave is followed by an afterwave, which is the giant U wave. The U wave is also visible in the limb leads. These giant U waves are characteristic of hypokalemia. The patient had a serum potassium of 1.1 mEq. per liter secondary to protracted diuretic therapy without potassium supplementation.

CASE STUDY 22: QUESTION

What is the rhythm? Long lead 2. The patient is a 67 year-old man admitted to the hospital with a history of having fainted suddenly.

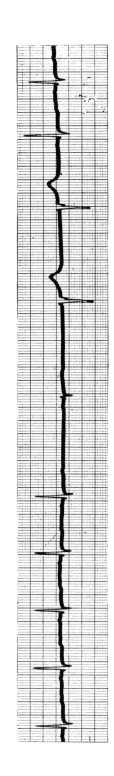

CASE STUDY 22: ANSWER

The first five beats are sinus beats with non-specific ST depression. Beat #6 is late, preceded by a P wave, and has a different QRS configuration. Beats #7 and 8 are not preceded by P waves, have a very aberrant QRS, and are ventricular escape beats. Beats #9 and 10 represent resumption of sinus rhythm. The altered configuration of beat #6 and the fact that it is preceded by a P wave suggests that this is a fusion beat, fusing the normally conducted QRS with the patient's ventricular escape mechanism. Further evidence that beat #6 is a fusion beat is the precise regularity of the R-R intervals between beats #6, 7 and 8. The marked slowing of the sinus rate with cessation of atrial activity indicates disease of the sinoatrial node. In view of the history of syncope, a permanent pacemaker is indicated.

NOTES

CASE STUDY 23: QUESTION

Standard chest leads (A) and chest lead taken one interspace above (B). What is the interpretation?

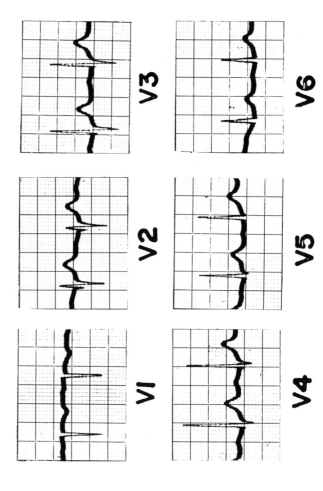

A

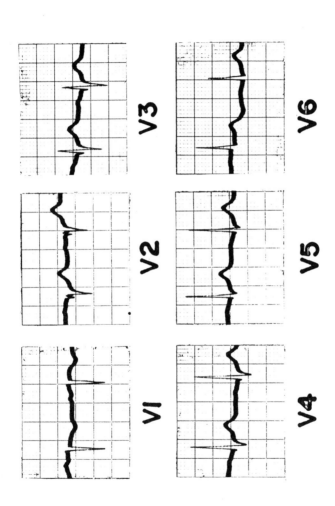

B

CASE STUDY 23: ANSWER

The standard V leads reveal a deep but narrow Q wave in V2. The T waves are normal. Such a Q wave is usually indicative of anteroseptal infarction. Leads taken one inter-space above or below the standard position may help to confirm this diagnosis. In B, leads taken one interspace above, there is a deep Q preceding a small r in V2 and a deep Q in V3 confirming the diagnosis of anteroseptal infarction.

CASE STUDY 24: QUESTION

What is the interpretation? Lead 2.

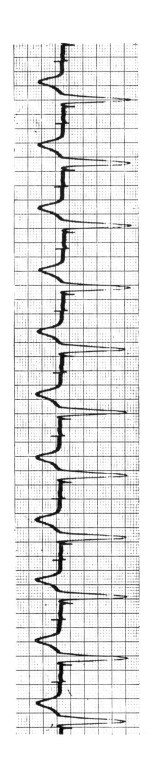

CASE STUDY 24: ANSWER

There are 2 pacemaker spikes visible at an interval of .22 second. The first activates the atrium producing a small positive wave. The second activates the ventricle. This patient has an atrial-ventricular synchronous pacemaker. There are two electrodes, one lies in the atrial appendage, the second in the right ventricle. These act in a synchronized fashion at a fixed sequential interval. Using this technique the atrial contribution to cardiac output is preserved independent of A-V conduction.

CASE STUDY 25: QUESTION

What is the rhythm? Rhythm strip obtained in a Coronary Care Unit from a patient with an acute myocardial infarction.

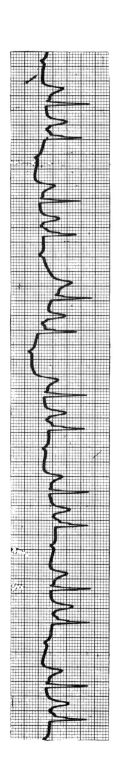

CASE STUDY 25: ANSWER

The rhythm is regular sinus rhythm with bigeminy due to frequent atrial premature contractions. This can be proven by careful examination of the ST segments of each beat. The premature beats are preceded by a P wave in the ST segment; the succeeding ST segments show no P wave. The P-R interval of the atrial premature contractions is .32 sec., whereas, the P-R interval of the sinus beat is .26 sec. The rhythm is regular sinus rhythm with 1° A-V block and premature atrial beats producing bigeminy. The P-R is further prolonged with the premature atrial contractions as the A-V junction is more refractory with the shorter cycle.

CASE STUDY 26: QUESTION

What is the interpretation? The patient is a 78 year-old man with long-standing hypertension and mild congestive failure.

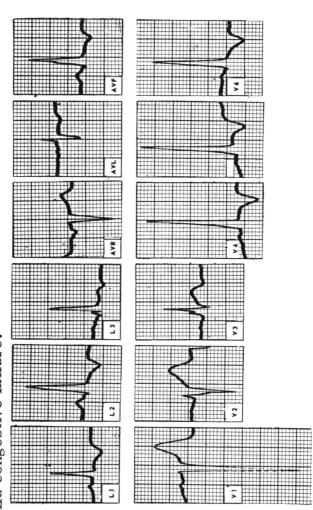

CASE STUDY 26: ANSWER

The rhythm is regular sinus rhythm. The electrical axis is $+75^\circ$. S-T is depressed with T inverted in leads 1, 2, AVL and V_6. S-T is slightly elevated with T inverted in 3, AVF, V_{3-5}. There is a deep S wave in V_1 and a tall R wave in V_4-V_6. The patient has evidence, on the basis of high precordial voltage, of left ventricular hypertrophy in a vertically placed heart. In this situation, the R wave is tall in 2, 3, and AVF. The S-T elevations suggest myocardial ischemia. Serial tracings should be obtained.

CASE STUDY 27: QUESTION

What is the rhythm? Lead V1.

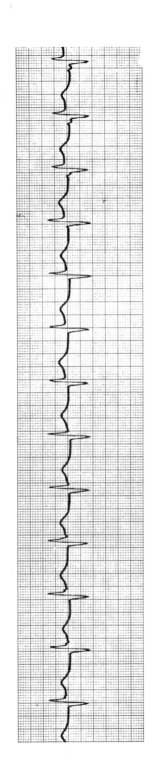

CASE STUDY 27: ANSWER

The rhythm is regular at approximately 72 beats/min. There are P waves visible in a varying relationship to the QRS. At the beginning of the record they are visible immediately following the R wave buried in the early portion of the S-T segment. The last three beats show the P wave preceding the QRS complex. However, the P-R interval is too short for these to be conducted beats and the R-R interval remains constant.

The rhythm is a junctional rhythm with a sinus rhythm at approximately the same rate. This is known as synchronization. There is no evidence of heart block. The rhythm may also be termed A-V dissociation without heart block.

NOTES

CASE STUDY 28: QUESTION

Standard ECG taken from a 74 year-old male admitted in congestive heart failure, receiving digitalis and diuretics. What is the diagnosis?

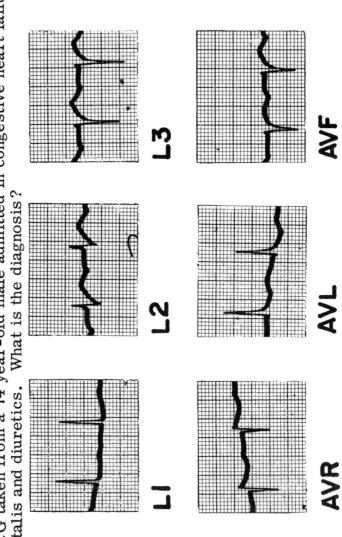

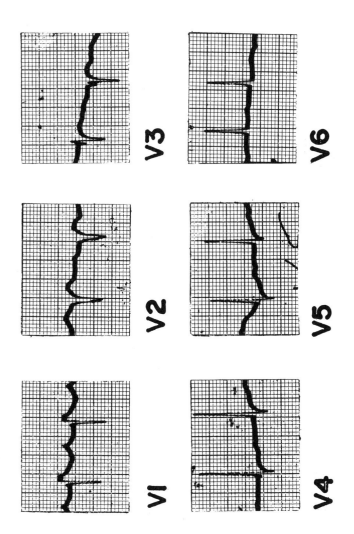

V3 V2 VI V6 V5 V4

CASE STUDY 28: ANSWER

P waves are not clearly seen in frontal plane leads. Atrial activity is seen between the QRS complexes in V1 and V2. The terminal portion of the QRS appears distorted and prolonged in these leads. This distortion is due to another P wave equidistant between the other clearly identifiable P waves. The rhythm is atrial tachycardia, at a rate of 192 with 2:1 heart block. In V6, the degree of block changes since the R-R interval is shorter. Atrial tachycardia with varying block is often a sign of digitalis toxicity.

There is a small r in V1, a Qs in V2, and a qr in V3 suggestive of anteroseptal infarction of indeterminate age.

NOTES

CASE STUDY 29: QUESTION

These two electrocardiograms were obtained on consecutive days. The patient had known coronary heart disease. What is the interpretation?

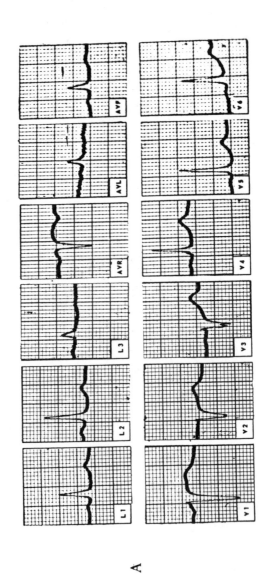

A

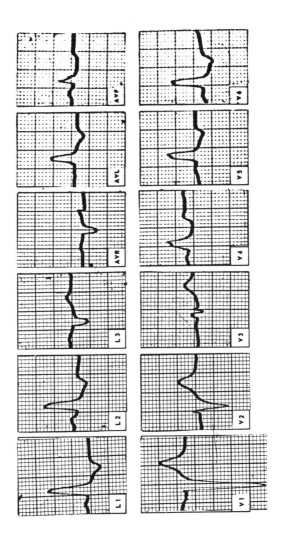

B

CASE STUDY 29: ANSWER

Tracing A shows regular sinus rhythm, with the QRS duration .11 sec. There is slight slurring of the S wave in V_3, and the initial portion of the R wave in V_4. There are no Q waves in leads 1, AVL, $V_{5\&6}$. The onset of the intrinsicoid deflection is delayed in these leads. The interpretation is incomplete left bundle branch block, a rather unusual electrocardiographic finding.

Tracing B confirms the diagnosis of left bundle branch disease, as it shows complete left bundle branch block. The QRS has widened to .13 sec., and the R waves are clearly more slurred. In addition, ST-T wave changes have developed of the type often seen with left bundle branch block.

CASE STUDY 30: QUESTION

ECG obtained from a 68 year-old woman admitted for gallbladder surgery. She had had diet-controlled diabetes and intermittent hypertension for many years. She was on no therapy. What is the interpretation?

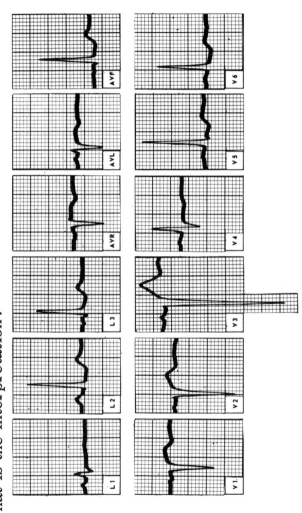

CASE STUDY 30: ANSWER

There is an Rs in lead 1. The mean electrical axis of the QRS is close to +90°. The mean electrical axis of the T wave is +75°. Lead V3 has a minute r wave smaller than the r in V2. The diminished initial positivity in V3 may be due to infarction of the anteroseptal region. The deep S wave in V3 (33 mm.) suggests large posteriorly directed forces (left ventricular). The tall R waves in V5 and deep S in V2 also suggest left ventricular hypertrophy. In keeping with this diagnosis are the depressed S-T segments with biphasic T waves in 3, AVF and V5-6.

The diagnosis is left ventricular hypertrophy in a patient with a vertical heart. In this situation, tall R waves appear in 2, 3 and AVF rather than 1 and AVL.

CASE STUDY 31: QUESTION

What is the rhythm? (Lead II)

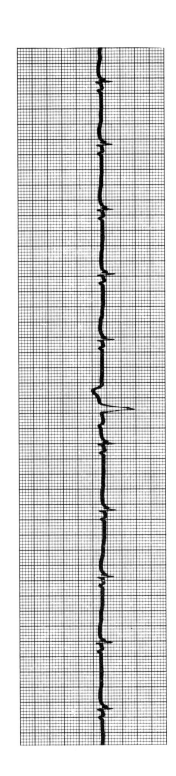

CASE STUDY 31: ANSWER

The rhythm is regular sinus rhythm at a rate of 70 beats/min. Beat #6 is premature and aberrant. Superficially it resembles a ventricular premature contraction. However, the T wave of the preceding QRS complex is deformed indicating that a P wave is superimposed. The P-R interval of this beat is slightly prolonged indicating a conduction delay due to increased refractoriness in A-V junctional tissue. The presence of an early P wave indicates that this is an atrial premature contraction with aberrant ventricular conduction. There is no compensatory pause. It is important to distinguish atrial from ventricular premature contractions as the therapeutic implications are different.

NOTES

CASE STUDY 32: QUESTION

This electrocardiogram was obtained from a 25 year-old asymptomatic man. What is the interpretation?

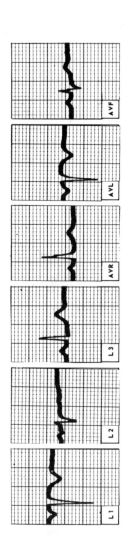

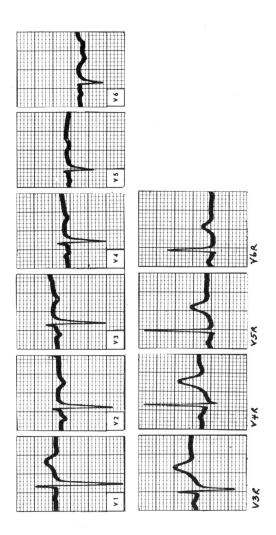

CASE STUDY 32: ANSWER

The P wave, QRS and T wave are negative in 1, as well as AVL. The V leads show loss of height of R wave in leads left of the sternum as well as negativity of the T wave. These changes are compatible with dextrocardia. V leads taken over the right precordium show normal R wave progression confirming the diagnosis.

If the RA and LA wires had been transposed accidentally, the standard leads would look like this patient's, but the V leads would be normal.

CASE STUDY 33: QUESTION

Continuous lead 2. What is the interpretation?

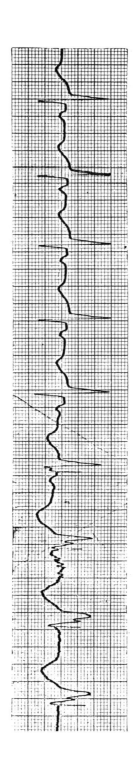

CASE STUDY 33: ANSWER

The first three beats are preceded by a pacemaker spike. The last five beats are preceded by P waves and the rhythm is regular sinus(with no pacemaker spike visible) at a very slightly more rapid rate. Beat #4 has a pacer spike preceding the QRS as well as a P wave. The QRS is intermediate in contour between the first three and the remaining beats. Beat #4 is, therefore, a fusion beat, with both P wave and pacer spike depolarizing the ventricle. The patient has a demand pacemaker which is suppressed when the spontaneous rate is adequate.

NOTES

CASE STUDY 34: QUESTION

The patient was a 37 year-old man with recent onset of fever and left pleuritic chest pain. What is the diagnosis?

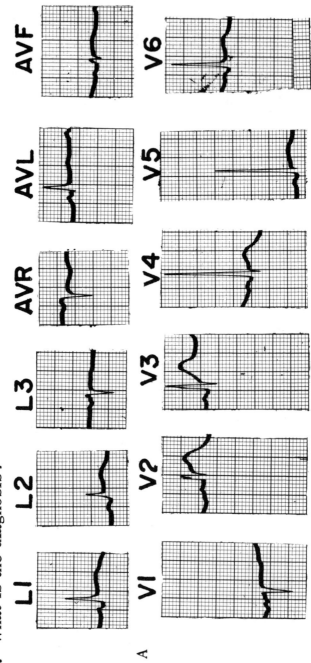

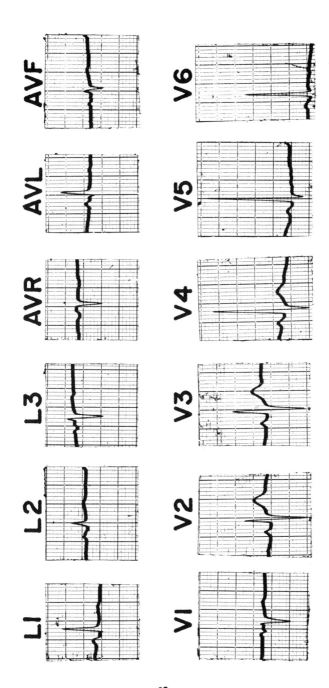

B

CASE STUDY 34: ANSWER

The rhythm is regular sinus. In leads 1, 2, AVL, AVF, and V2 to V6, S-T segments are moderately elevated. These findings are strongly suggestive of pericarditis. They may occur in patients as a normal variant, so serial tracings are necessary to confirm the diagnosis. Tracing B obtained 1 week later shows an isoelectric S-T segment with flat T waves, particularly apparent in V5 and V6. These changes are consistent with the diagnosis of acute pericarditis.

CASE STUDY 35: QUESTION

Lead V_1. The patient was a 28 year-old man complaining of palpitations. There were no auscultatory abnormalities and he had a normal chest X-ray. What is the electro-cardiographic diagnosis?

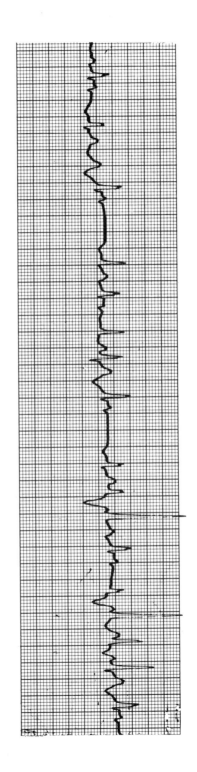

CASE STUDY 35: ANSWER

The P waves vary in configuration and are grossly irregular in rate. Beats #4 and 7 have a narrow QRS but are aberrantly conducted. The rhythm has been termed chaotic atrial arrhythmia, or multifocal atrial tachycardia. It is often seen in patients with end-stage pulmonary disease, but occasionally occurs in normal individuals.

CASE STUDY 36: QUESTION

What is the interpretation? Lead 1.

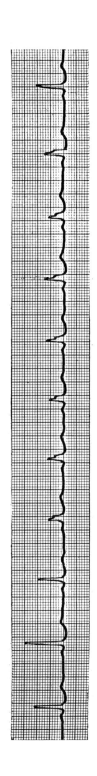

CASE STUDY 36: ANSWER

The rhythm is regular sinus rhythm with slight variation in rate. The first three beats show the QRS duration of .10 second with slight variations in form. The ensuing beats have a QRS duration of .14 second with a markedly aberrant QRS. The final beat again shows a narrowed QRS. The aberrant beats are left bundle branch block, and occur when the rate accelerates from 64 to 69. This is, therefore, a rate-dependent left bundle branch block.

NOTES

CASE STUDY 37: QUESTION

Tracings of a 46 year-old male admitted with recurrent chest pain. ECG taken 8/28 (A) was taken shortly after admission. The tracing of 8/29 (B) was taken following a bout of prolonged severe chest pain. What is the interpretation?

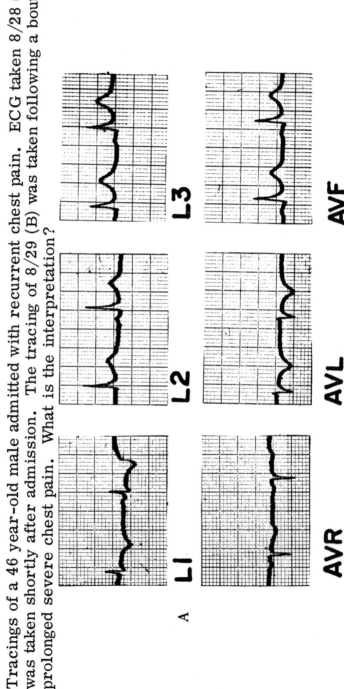

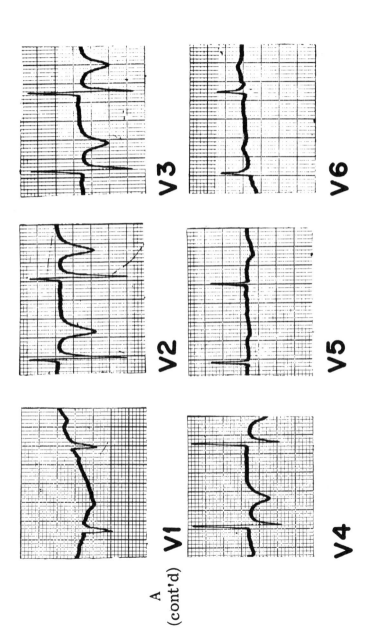

A
(cont'd)

V1 V2 V3

V4 V5 V6

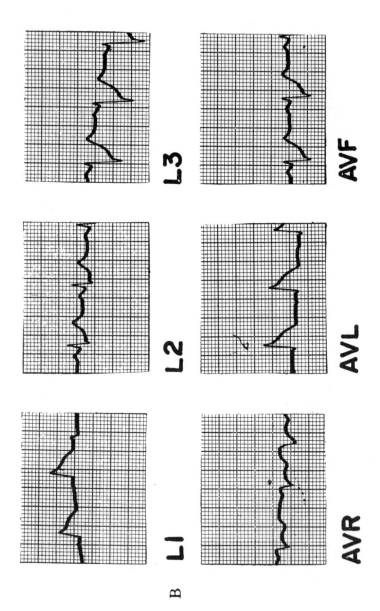

L3

AVF

L2

AVL

B   LI

AVR

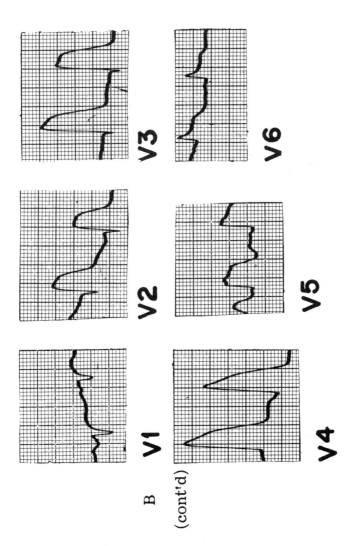

B
(cont'd)

V1 V2 V3

V4 V5 V6

CASE STUDY 37: ANSWER

ECG on 8/28 shows regular sinus rhythm. There are symmetrically inverted T waves in lead 1, AVL, V2 through V4. These changes are compatible with an acute myocardial infarction, or coronary insufficiency. On 8/29 there is marked elevation of the ST segment in leads, 1, AVL, V2 through V6, with a Q wave in V2 and V3. There is reciprocal depression of the ST segment in II, III and AVF. These new changes are indicative of a fresh through and through infarction of the anterior wall.

CASE STUDY 38: QUESTION

What is the rhythm ? (lead 2)

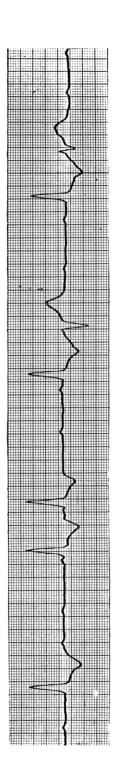

The atrial rate is 95 and no P waves conduct to the ventricle. Therefore, the patient has complete heart block. The ventricular rhythm is irregular and slow. After beats number 2, 4, and 6, there are premature beats which vary in QRS configuration, but occur at approximately the same coupling interval. The first of these coupled beats is identical to the usual idioventricular beat. The fixed coupling suggests that each of these beats arises in a fixed focus, but conducts through the ventricle via different pathways.

CASE STUDY 39: QUESTION

What is the diagnosis? The electrocardiogram was obtained from a 53 year-old woman with symptoms of increasing shortness of breath of several years duration and heart murmur known for at least 25 years.

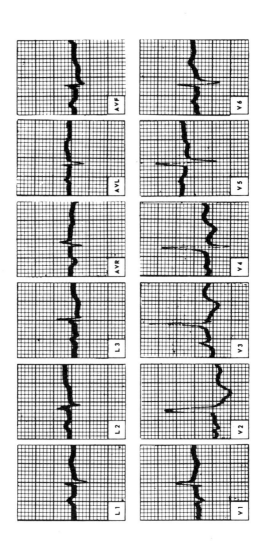

The rhythm is sinus; the P wave is biphasic, with a broad negative component in lead V1, and tall and narrow in V3. The axis is right at approximately 100°. There is a tendency to low voltage. In the right sided precordial leads, V1 and V2, there is a tall R wave preceded by a small q. The right axis deviation and tall right sided R waves are evidence of right ventricular hypertrophy. In addition, the P in V1 suggests left atrial enlargement and the tall P in V3 is suggestive of right atrial enlargement, as well. These findings are consistent with right ventricular hypertrophy and bi-atrial enlargement. They are often seen in mitral stenosis accompanied by significant pulmonary hypertension, as was the case in this patient.

CASE STUDY 40: QUESTION

What is the rhythm? (Lead 2)

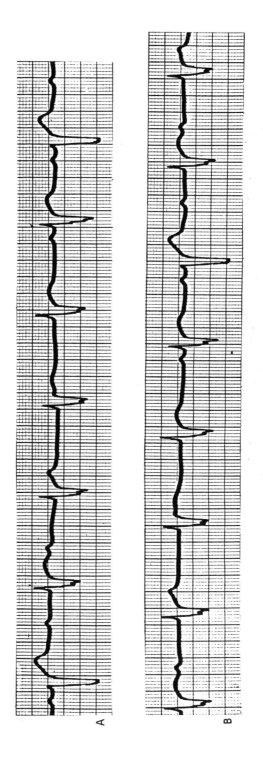

Strip A shows regular sinus activity with an atrial rate of 64 and many of the P waves noncounducted or buried in the QRS complexes. P wave #2 is followed by a long PR interval of 0.48 sec. and QRS complex #2 is more aberrant and differing in form from beat #1. The succeeding three QRS complexes resemble beat #2 and are perfectly regular at a rate of 56. They are unrelated to the preceding P waves. Beat #6 has a PR interval of .19 sec. and is intermediate in form. Beat #7 resembles beat #1 and is preceded by a normal PR interval of 0.20 sec. This represents second degree heart block with an idioventricular escape rhythm occurring where the P waves are not conducted. Beat #6 is a fusion beat being intermediate in form. Strip B shows further confirmation of this phenomenon. The initial impression of a Wenckebach phenomenon, as manifest by gradually increasing PR intervals, is clearly not the case in view of the change in QRS form and its precise regularity. In all likelihood, this represents a Mobitz II type block since the conducted P-R intervals are precisely regular and the QRS of the conducted beats is widened to 0.16 sec. More protracted observations of the rhythm would be necessary to confirm this. His bundle electrocardiography at times would be of value in proving that the block was below the bundle of His rather than in the AV node.

CASE STUDY 41: QUESTION

The patient was a 39 year-old man with a history of a murmur since infancy, but no symptomatology or significant prior history. What is the interpretation?

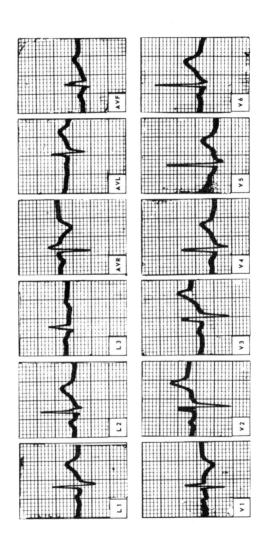

CASE STUDY 41: ANSWER

The rhythm is regular sinus rhythm. The QRS duration is .10 sec. There is an rsR' pattern in V1, which occurs in the presence of an atrial septal defect. The pattern is identical to incomplete right bundle branch block. It would rarely be normal in this age group. With large atrial septal defects, there is often enlargement of the right atrium and P wave abnormalities. This was not the case in this patient. He had a small hemodynamically rather insignificant atrial septal defect which was not considered adequate reason for surgical intervention. He was allowed to continue normal activity without restriction.

NOTES

CASE STUDY 42: QUESTION   108

What is the diagnosis? The patient was a 60 year-old man. The initial tracing was tak-
en on a routine examination. The subsequent tracing was taken one year later when he
had been admitted to the hospital with acute chest pain.

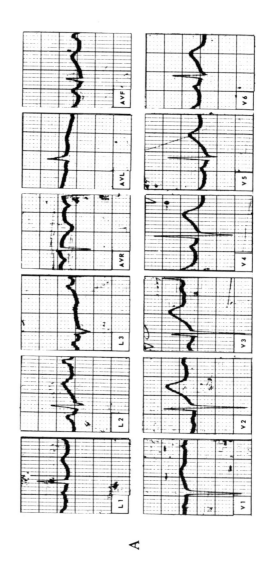

A

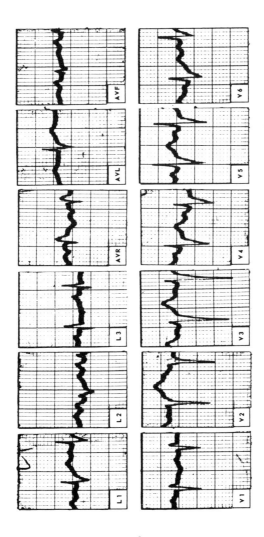

B

Tracing A demonstrates regular sinus rhythm with a perfectly normal electrocardiogram. Tracing B shows the development of a slurred S wave in lead 1, small Q_3 and AVF and terminal R wave in leads AVR and V_1. The QRS duration is 0.11 sec. The patient has developed incomplete right bundle branch block with increased clockwise rotation as manifest by the poor R wave progression in the precordial leads to V_5. These changes are highly suspicious of acute cor pulmonale. The diagnosis of pulmonary emboli was confirmed by lung scan.

CASE STUDY 43: QUESTION

What is the rhythm? The patient is a 52 year-old man with an acute myocardial infarction. This is lead 2.

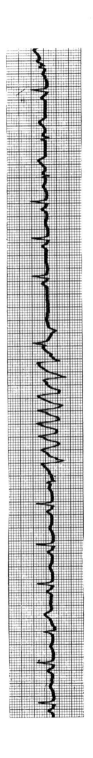

CASE STUDY 43: ANSWER

The first two beats show regular sinus rhythm and are followed by a ventricular premature contraction occurring late after the T wave. Beat #6 is followed by a ventricular premature contraction falling on the downstroke of the T wave and is followed immediately by a burst of chaotic ventricular activity. These ventricular beats are grossly irregular and vary in form. The ventricular arrhythmia stops spontaneously and regular sinus rhythm resumes with occasional ventricular premature contractions occurring after the T wave. This rhythm is a rather "well-organized" form of ventricular fibrillation. It is occasionally referred to as ventricular flutter. This arrhythmia may eventuate in persistent ventricular fibrillation, and therefore requires aggressive therapy.

An alternative explanation of this arrhythmia is that it has a supraventricular origin with aberrant ventricular conduction. This is unlikely in view of the presence of ventricular premature beats, the irregular rhythm and the ventricular rate of 300 beats/minute.

CASE STUDY 44: QUESTION

What is the rhythm? (Lead 2).

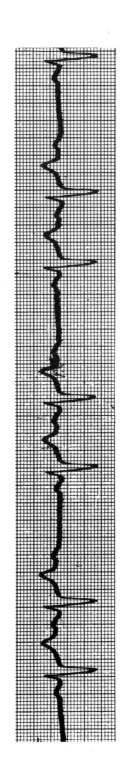

CASE STUDY 44: ANSWER

The PR interval of the first two complexes is normal at 0.20 sec. The QRS duration is .16 sec. The third P wave is nonconducted. This cycle recurs in the remainder of the strip. This is second degree heart block of the Mobitz Type II variety. Note the wide QRS. When this type of heart block develops, either de novo or in the course of an acute myocardial infarction, a cardiac pacemaker is usually recommended as the incidence of complete heart block is high in this situation. In contradistinction to Mobitz I, the block is usually below the bundle of His, in the bundle branches.

CASE STUDY 45: QUESTION

This electrocardiogram was obtained from a 20 year-old male admitted for elective repair of a hernia. He was asymptomatic. What is the interpretation?

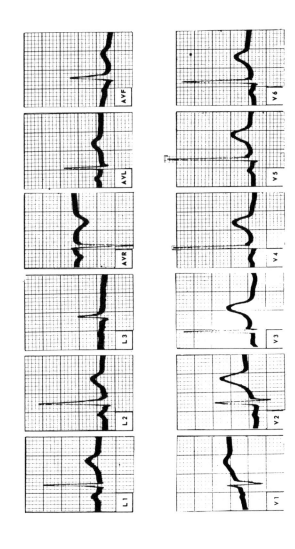

The rhythm is sinus. The S-T segment is slightly elevated in V2-V6. The J point is above the isoelectric line; the S-T segment is convex downward. Such elevation of the S-T segment is usually a normal variant and is frequently seen in young people. It is often called early repolarization. In addition there is marked counterclockwise rotation of the QRS in the horizontal plane. This is manifested by the tall R wave in V2-V6; the transition zone is between V1 and V2. This is a normal phenomenon.

CASE STUDY 46: QUESTION

Continuous strip lead 2. What is the rhythm?

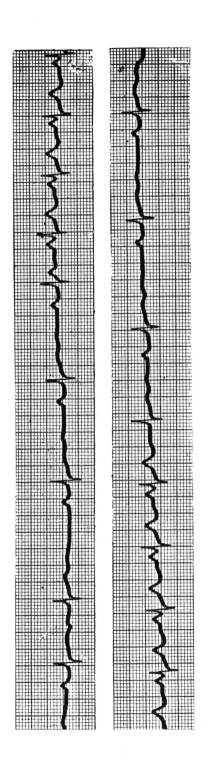

CASE STUDY 46: ANSWER

The first beat is sinus in origin with a P-R interval of .30 second. The second QRS is preceded by an inverted P wave. This is an atrial premature beat, also with P-R prolongation. There are then three sinus beats at a rate of 52, with a prolonged P-R interval. After the fifth QRS complex the atrial rate accelerates to 165 beats per minute with 2 to 1 atrioventricular block. During the tachycardia all T waves appear peaked, suggesting that a P wave is superimposed. The last three beats in the second strip show sinus bradycardia at a rate of 47 beats per minute with a prolonged P-R interval.

The fifth QRS in strip 2 is followed by a T wave resembling the T wave of beats #6, 7 and 8. The P wave preceding beat #5 is superimposed on the T wave of beat #4 and is conducted with a P-R of .46 second. This proves that during the tachycardia the P wave immediately preceding the QRS is not the conducted one.

A slow supraventricular rhythm alternating with a rapid one is called a bradytachyarrhythmia. It is often associated with A-V conduction disturbances, manifested in this case by prolongation of the P-R interval. Treatment to speed the sinus rhythm is rarely effective. Often a pacemaker is needed to prevent recurrent tachycardia. If bouts of rapid rhythm persist, agents such as digitalis, quinidine or propranolol may then be used safely.

CASE STUDY 47: QUESTION

What is the interpretation? Lead 2.

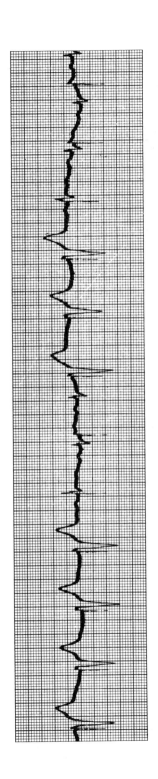

A pacer spike precedes the first four beats and depolarizes the ventricle. The pacer spike precedes the fifth beat but the QRS is relatively normal in configuration. A P wave is present before this beat. The sixth beat is a sinus beat followed by a pacer spike. The next three beats are paced (the pacer spike captures the ventricle). The eleventh beat is a fusion between the normally conducted QRS and ventricular depolarization due to the pacemaker discharge. The last three beats are sinus with pacer spikes not related to the QRS complexes.

If the patient has a fixed rate pacemaker, it is functioning properly. The sinus node and the pacer spike alternately control ventricular depolarization. The pacer spike is regular and appears whether or not spontaneous beats occur. If the pacemaker is a demand type it is malfunctioning as it fails to shut off during spontaneous depolarization.

A knowledge of the type of pacemaker is essential for proper interpretation.

CASE STUDY 48: QUESTION

57 year-old man admitted for prostatic surgery; what is the diagnosis?

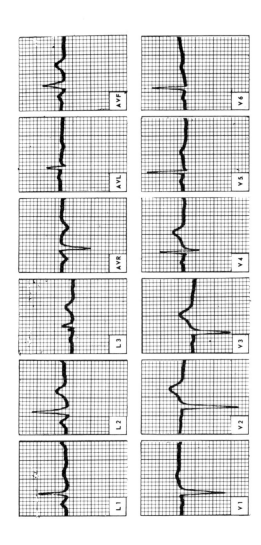

CASE STUDY 48: ANSWER

There is failure of R wave progression in V1-3, with the T wave positive in these leads. This finding could represent an old anteroseptal infarction. However, many patients with similar electrocardiograms have been demonstrated to be free of coronary artery disease and infarction. T3 is taller than T1 and the T in VL is inverted. These are non-specific abnormalities.

CASE STUDY 49: QUESTION

This electrocardiogram was obtained from a 68 year-old male who had chronic short-ness of breath. He had been a heavy smoker for many years.

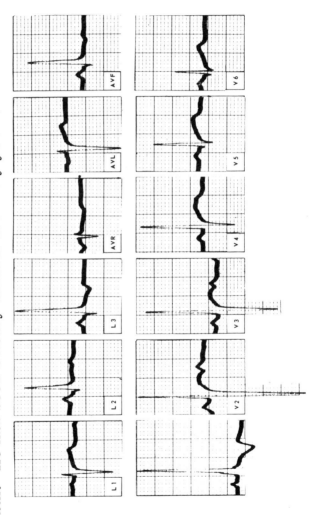

The rhythm is sinus. The QRS is 0.10 sec. in duration. The mean electrical axis of the QRS in the frontal plane is to the right at +105°. The T wave is negative in 3 and AVF. There is a large R wave in V1 of 27 mv. A small q, large R and small s are present in V6. The P waves are peaked in 2, 3 and AVF.

The most likely diagnosis is right ventricular hypertrophy based on the marked right axis deviation and the large R in V1. The QRS configuration in the frontal plane resembles left posterior hemiblock – but this diagnosis cannot be made in the presence of right ventricular hypertrophy. The QRS is too narrow to diagnose complete right bundle branch block. X-ray of the chest demonstrated the presence of right ventricular hypertrophy.

CASE STUDY 50: QUESTION

Lead 2 - What is the rhythm?

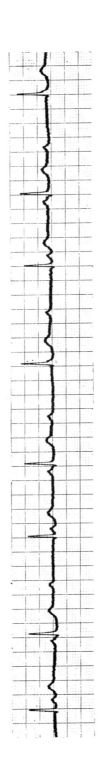

The P waves are regular at a rate of 75/min. Not all P waves are followed by R waves. The R-R interval is irregular. The interval between the QRS complexes of beats 2 and 3, 4 and 5, 5 and 6, and 7 and 8 is the same at 1.4 seconds. The second, fourth and seventh QRS complexes occur earlier and all have a P wave preceding them at an interval of .14 second. The rhythm is high grade A-V block with intermittent capture of the ventricle by the atrium.

CASE STUDY 51: QUESTION

The patient is a 43 year-old female with a long history of rheumatic heart disease. What is the interpretation?

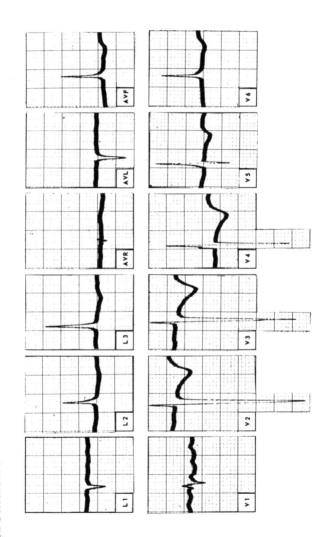

The rhythm is atrial fibrillation; P waves are not seen but fibrillatory waves are present.

The mean electrical axis in the frontal plane is +120°. The R wave in V1 is almost equal to the S wave. Deep S waves are present in V2 and V3. A prominent R wave is again in V6.

The marked right axis deviation as well as a large R in V1 suggest right ventricular hypertrophy. A lead V3R to the right of V1 did show an R greater than S confirming the diagnosis. The presence of a deep S in V2 and V3 plus a large R in V6 is consistent with left ventricular hypertrophy. This electrocardiogram is compatible with combined ventricular hypertrophy.

CASE STUDY 52: QUESTION

What is the rhythm? (Lead 2)

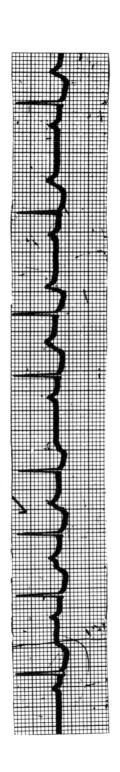

The initial four complexes demonstrate progressive prolongation of the PR interval. The PR interval of the first beat is 0.14 sec. The PR interval of beat #4 is .32 sec. and the P wave is superimposed on the preceding T wave. The following P wave (P #5) is buried in the S-T segment of beat #4 and is not conducted. The next P wave again has a short PR and the cycle recurs. The final two complexes represent classic 2:1 heartblock with a P wave buried in the T of complex of #7. This is second degree AV block (Mobitz I) with Wenckebach periods. In patients with second degree AV block, Wenckebach periods and narrow QRS, the conduction delay is usually in the AV node.

CASE STUDY 53: QUESTION

What is the rhythm? Tracing was obtained from a patient being monitored in the CCU.

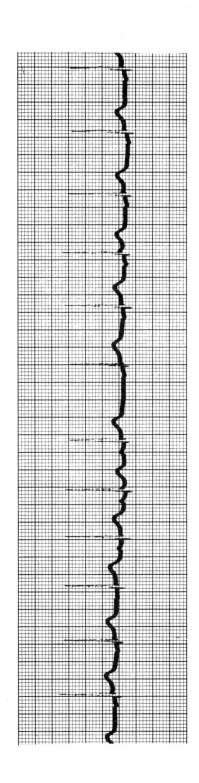

CASE STUDY 53: ANSWER

Each QRS is preceded by a P wave which varies in configuration and polarity. The rhythm is grossly irregular. Diagnosis is wandering atrial pacemaker. Usually this arrhythmia has no clinical significance. It may represent disease of the sino-atrial node.

CASE STUDY 54: QUESTION

66 year-old man admitted with congestive failure receiving digitalis. See figures A and B on the following pages. Figure A was obtained on admission. Figure B was taken 3 days later after further digitalis therapy. The manifestations of failure had increased. What is the electrocardiographic interpretation? Should the digitalis dose be increased, decreased or remain unchanged?

134

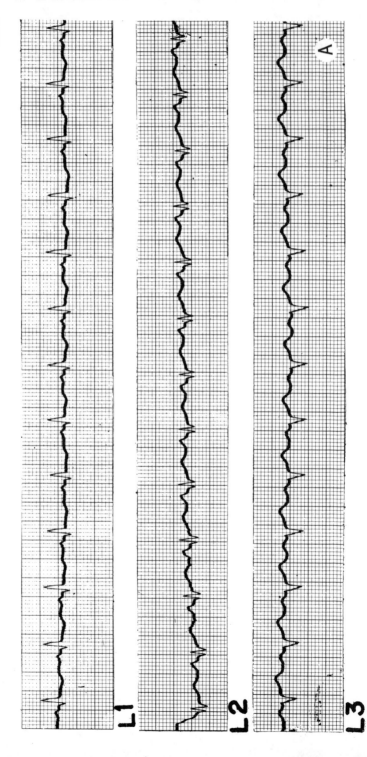

L1

L2

L3

A

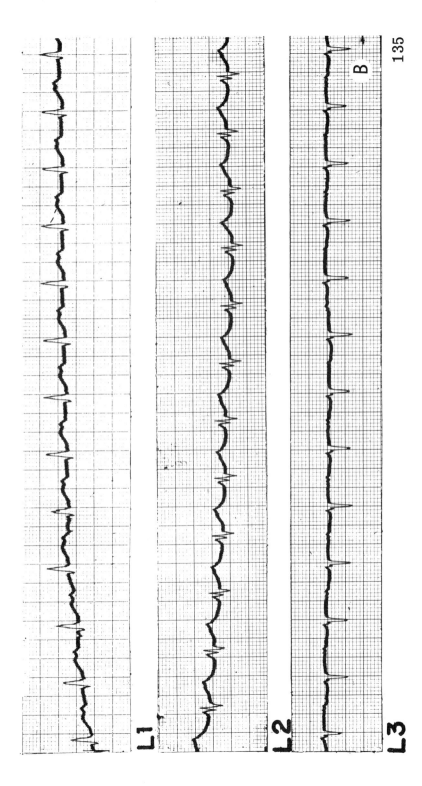

L1

L2

B

L3

135

A - This record shows sinus tachycardia at a rate of 100. Q waves are visible in lead 1 and 2 and T is inverted in lead 1.

B - The rhythm has changed to atrial tachycardia at a rate of 185 with 2:1 block. Alternative P waves are superimposed on the T wave and the initial portion of the QRS. The QRS in lead 2 is deformed by the P wave, masking the Q wave. This rhythm is evidence of digitalis toxicity and the drug should be stopped.

CASE STUDY 55: QUESTION

This electrocardiogram was obtained 1 year after a myocardial infarction. The patient is asymptomatic. What is the interpretation?

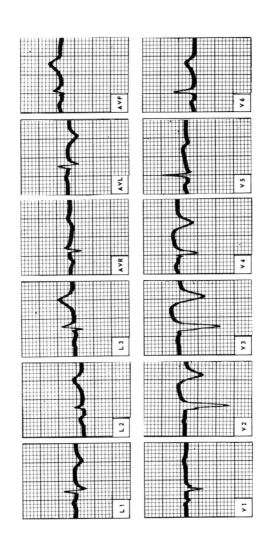

The rhythm is sinus. The voltage of the QRS is low and less than 5 mv. in the frontal plane leads and less than 15 mv. in the precordial leads. The T wave is inverted in 1 and AVL. A QS complex with elevated ST segments and negative T wave is present in V1-3. A qrS complex with negative T is seen in V4. The T is biphasic in V5.

These changes are compatible with an anteroseptal infarction. The persistent ST seg-ment elevations in complexes with an abnormal QS suggest a ventricular aneurysm of the anterior wall of the left ventricle.

NOTES

What is the interpretation of this electrocardiogram obtained from a 78 year-old man with a history of episodes of syncope ?

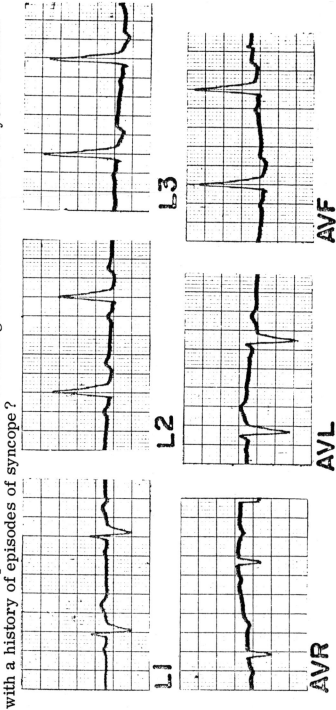

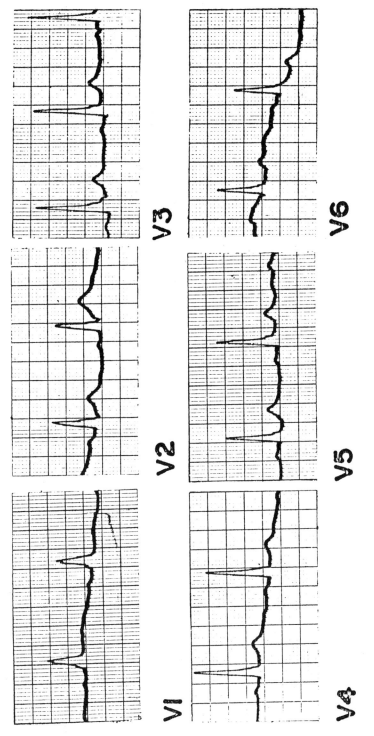

V1 V2 V3 V4 V5 V6

141

CASE STUDY 56: ANSWER

The tracing shows regular sinus rhythm with right axis deviation ($> 100^\circ$) as indicated by a small r wave in lead 1, tall R waves in leads 2, 3 and AVF. There are small q waves in leads 2, 3 and AVF. The QRS measures .14 sec. In V_1, the tall slurred R wave is evidence of right bundle branch block. The patient has right axis deviation with right bundle branch block. In an elderly patient without right ventricular enlargement, this pattern is evidence of disease of the right bundle and the posterior fascicle of the left bundle. This situation is often accompanied by transient heart block or the development of permanent heart block and, in a patient with a history of syncope, indicates the need for a cardiac pacemaker.

CASE STUDY 57: QUESTION

What is the rhythm? Lead 2.

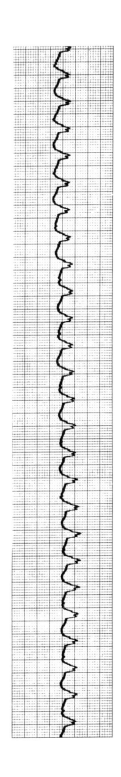

CASE STUDY 57: ANSWER

The QRS complexes are aberrant and the QRS duration is 0.16 sec. The rate is 145 beats/min. and is precisely regular. Following every alternate QRS there is a notch on the T wave. This probably represents atrial activity and, since it is related in a fixed fashion to the QRS, it probably represents retrograde activation of the atrium after alternate QRS complexes. The rhythm is, therefore, ventricular tachycardia with 2 to 1 ventriculo-atrial block.

CASE STUDY 58: QUESTION

Lead 2. This record was obtained from a 78 year-old male with advanced renal disease. What is the interpretation?

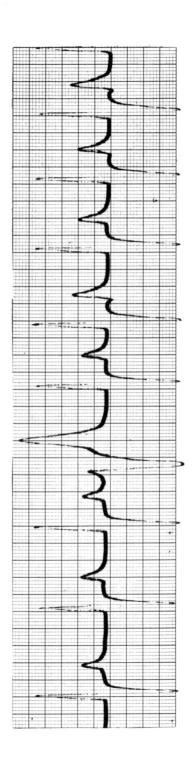

CASE STUDY 58: ANSWER

No atrial activity is detected. The ventricular rate is slightly irregular. Beat #4 is a ventricular premature contraction. The T waves are tall and markedly peaked.

This type of T wave is characteristic of hyperkalemia as is absence of visible atrial activity. The patient's serum potassium level was 8.2 mgm%.

CASE STUDY 59: QUESTION

What is the rhythm? The patient is receiving digitalis and has chronic congestive heart failure.

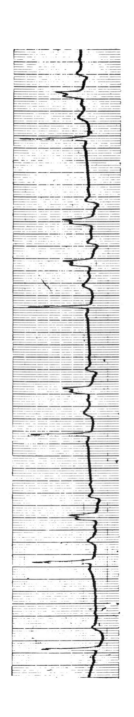

CASE STUDY 59: ANSWER

The rhythm is regular sinus rhythm at a rate of 85 a minute. The 2nd, 5th, 8th, 12th and 15th P waves are non-conducted. The 3rd, 5th, 7th, 8th, and 10th QRS shows a left bundle branch block pattern with a PR interval identical to the normally conducted beats (#1, 2, 4, 6, and 9). This is rate related left bundle branch block in a patient with varying heart block (Mobitz II). This is not the Wenckebach phenomenon as the PR interval is constant. Heart block of this type may be secondary to digitalis toxicity or disease of the conduction system. Digitalis should be discontinued, and if the block persists, insertion of a permanent pacemaker should be considered.

CASE STUDY 60: QUESTION

What is the diagnosis? The patient was a 37 year-old woman with a vague history of palpitations but no other specific symptoms.

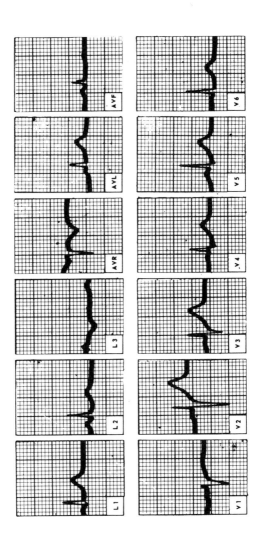

CASE STUDY 60: ANSWER

The rhythm is regular sinus rhythm. The PR interval is 0.09 sec. and there is an extremely short PR segment. This is most clearly seen in the precordial leads V4 to V6. The QRS duration is 0.08 sec. The patient has the syndrome of the short PR interval with a normal QRS (Lown-Ganong-Levine Syndrome). Such patients, while often asymptomatic, may have bouts of supraventricular arrhythmias. The condition is usually benign and is only rarely accompanied by significant cardiac pathology.

CASE STUDY 61: QUESTION

What is the rhythm? Lead 2. The patient was a 78 year-old man complaining of inter-mittent dizzy spells.

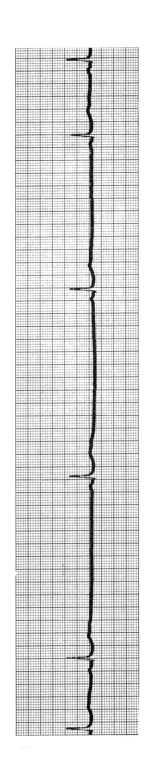

CASE STUDY 61: ANSWER

The first two beats are of sinus origin at a rate of approximately 60 beats/min. The rate then slows to approximately 25 beats/min. This is marked sinus bradycardia and prob- ably was the cause of the dizzy spells. Patients with symptomatic sinus bradycardia re- spond poorly to drugs and are benefited by pacemaker therapy.

CASE STUDY 62: QUESTION

The patient is a 66 year-old woman with a long history of coronary artery disease. What is the interpretation of this electrocardiogram?

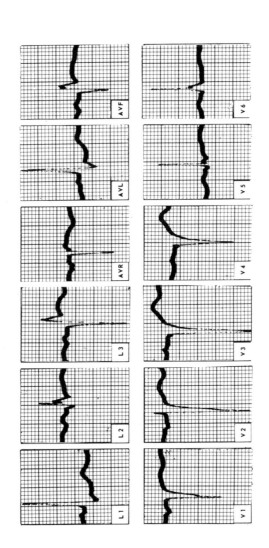

The rhythm is sinus. There is a deep Q wave in 2, 3, and AVF. There is depression of the ST segment in 1, AVL and elevation in 2, 3, AVF. A QS complex is present in V1 and rS in V2. A QS complex is again present in V3 and V4 with notching of the initial downstroke. The shift from a QS to rS and then QS in the precordial leads is indicative of anterior wall myocardial infarction. The initial notching of the downstroke of the QS in V3 and V4 is confirmatory evidence.

The abnormal Q wave in leads 2, 3, and AVF are evidence of inferior wall myocardial infarction. The patient, therefore, has multiple myocardial infarctions. The age of the infarctions cannot be determined from a single tracing. The elevated ST segments in 2, 3, and AVF may be a sign of recent inferior wall infarction, but serial tracings would be necessary to confirm this diagnosis. Persistent ST segment elevations in these leads may indicate an inferior wall aneurysm.

CASE STUDY 63: QUESTION

The patient is a 69 year-old male admitted following a syncopal episode. The electro-cardiogram was obtained on admission. What is the interpretation?

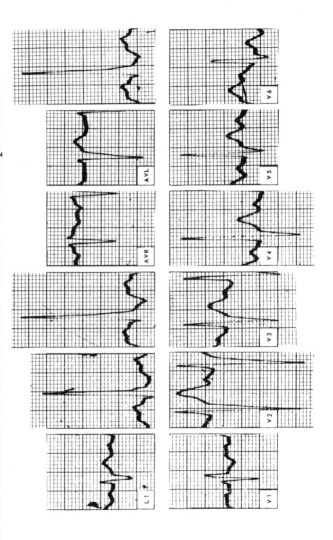

CASE STUDY 63: ANSWER

The rhythm is sinus tachycardia with a PR interval of 0.18 sec. The QRS is widened to 0.12 sec. There is an rSR' in V1 and a qRS in V6 compatible with right bundle branch block. In the frontal plane, there is marked right axis deviation (+100°) with an rS in 1, and a qR in 3. These latter changes indicate the presence of left posterior hemiblock (LPH - fascicular block). When LPH is present with right bundle branch block and the patient has a history of syncope, a permanent pacemaker should be implanted.

CASE STUDY 64: QUESTION

What is the rhythm? (V1)

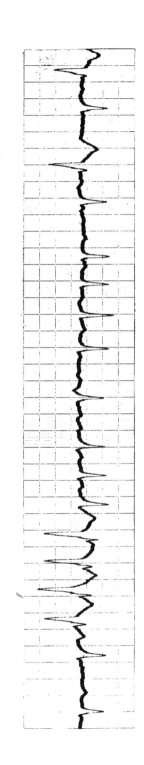

The ventricular rate is grossly irregular and the rhythm is atrial fibrillation. Beats 3-7 are aberrantly conducted with a regular R-R interval and two similar beats occur at the end of the tracing. The coupling interval of the aberrant beats is identical. The differential as to the origin of these beats is either ventricular premature contractions with a burst of ventricular tachycardia or aberrantly conducted supraventricular beats. Many of the normally conducted beats have a short R-R interval and are not aberrantly conducted. This suggests that the aberrant beats may arise in a lower ventricular focus and represent ventricular irritability. The alternate possibility is the Ashman phenomenon. This occurs when a short R-R interval follows a long R-R interval. In this situation, the beat following the pause is normally conducted. There is aberration of the succeeding beat with the short interval. These aberrant beats often have a right bundle branch block configuration and their initial .04 sec. resembles the beats with aberration as in this case.

The only means of absolute differentiation is to obtain a His bundle recording. If the His spike precedes the aberrant QRS it would prove the supraventricular origin of the beat.

NOTES

What is the diagnosis? The patient was a 29 year-old woman with a history of repeated episodes of fainting usually occurring following strenuous exertion. Her son, age nine, had similar symptoms.

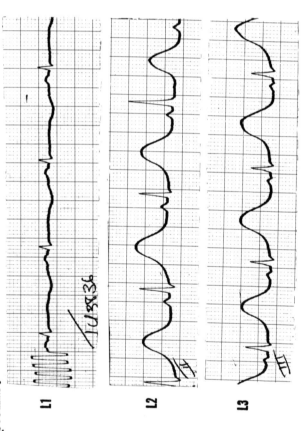

L1

L2

L3

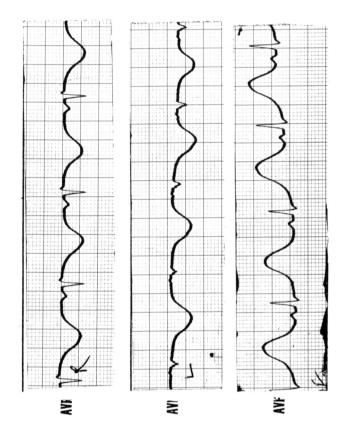

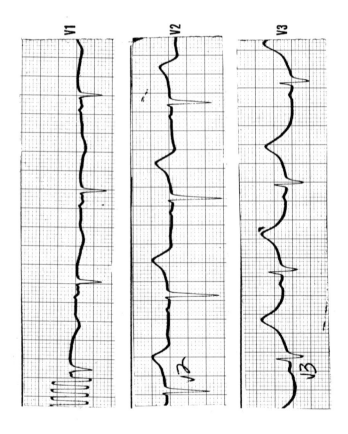

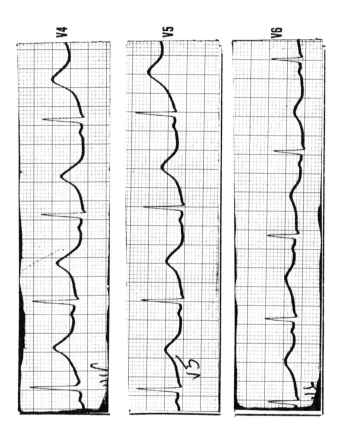

CASE STUDY 65: ANSWER

The electrocardiogram shows unique QT prolongation with the QT measuring 0.62 sec. These bizarre prolongations were variable in this patient and at times the QT appeared almost normal. Such marked changes in the QT interval occurring in a patient with syncopal seizures has been termed the syndrome of the prolonged QT interval and has often terminated fatally due to ventricular fibrillation. Attempts at control with medications such as dilantin or propranolol have been of variable value. There have been reports of patients successfully treated with cervical sympathectomy. The syndrome is often accompanied by deafness, and is heritable.

CASE STUDY 66: QUESTION

The patient is a 52 year-old woman known to have had rheumatic heart disease, atrial fibrillation and congestive failure, who is receiving diuretics and digitalis. She is admitted for increasing heart failure. Lead II was taken on admission. What is the diagnosis?

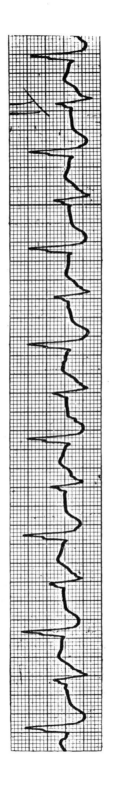

CASE STUDY 66: ANSWER

The rhythm is regular and rapid, at a rate of 118/min. Atrial activity is not discernible. The QRS complex alternates in form from beat to beat. This rhythm is called bidirectional junctional tachycardia. It is almost always due to digitalis toxicity.

When a patient with atrial fibrillation on digitalis develops a regular rhythm, the drug must be stopped and an electrocardiogram taken to determine the nature of the new rhythm.

CASE STUDY 67: QUESTION

Lead 2. What is the rhythm?

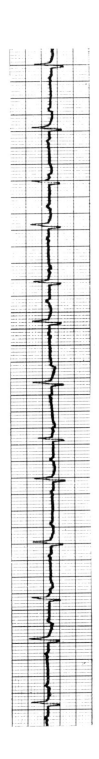

167

CASE STUDY 67: ANSWER

P waves are present at a rate of 155/min. and are regular. A P wave precedes the first QRS with a P-R interval of .16 sec. The second P wave is blocked. The third P wave is conducted with a P-R interval of .16 sec. The fourth P wave is conducted with a P-R interval of 0.26 sec. The fifth P wave is blocked. The process is then repeated. This is second degree heart block, Mobitz type I (Wenckebach periods), with 2:1 alternating with 3:2 A-V block. The atrial mechanism is probably atrial tachycardia.

CASE STUDY 68: QUESTION

This 66 year-old woman, in generally good health, was admitted for pre-operative evaluation prior to an elective surgical procedure. What is the interpretation of this electrocardiogram?

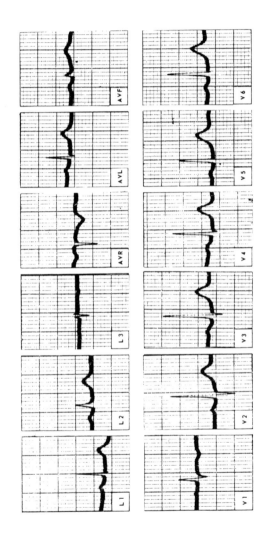

CASE STUDY 68: ANSWER

The rhythm is regular sinus; the standard limb leads are within normal limits. In V1, the R wave is 5 mv. in height. The S wave is small. The remainder of the V leads are normal. The finding of an isolated dominant R wave in V1 is suspicious of old postero-lateral infarction, as this rarely occurs in normal individuals. While this tracing does not conclusively indicate old damage, it is strongly suspicious. Right ventricular hyper-trophy can produce a large R wave in V1, but is usually accompanied by right axis devi-ation of at least 100°.

NOTES

The patient was an 84 year-old man with heart block and a ventricular synchronous pacemaker had been inserted. The top strip was obtained shortly afterward. The middle strip was taken six months after insertion at an emergency room following a syncopal episode. The bottom strip was obtained the next day following another syncopal episode. What is the interpretation?

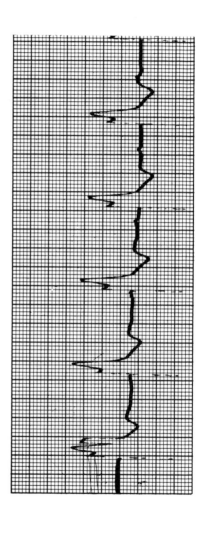

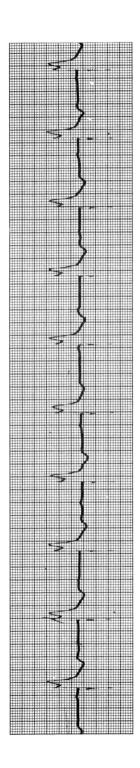
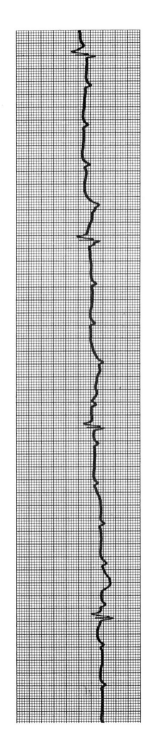

CASE STUDY 69: ANSWER

The top strip shows a regular pacemaker spike at a rate of 70/min. Each spike is followed by a ventricular depolarization. The pacer is functioning properly in a fixed rate mode.

The middle strip shows regular pacer spikes – each followed by ventricular depolarization. However, the rate of the pacemaker has decreased to 55/min.

The bottom strip shows complete heart block at a rate of 21/min. A spike is superimposed on each spontaneous QRS.

Sudden slowing of the escape rate of a demand pacemaker – or the fixed rate of a fixed rate pacemaker of over 2 beats/min. – indicates impending pacemaker failure. The patient should have the pacemaker pack changed. This was not done in this case at the time of the second strip.

CASE STUDY 70: QUESTION

The patient is a 72 year-old man with a history of previous myocardial infarctions. He was admitted to the Coronary Care Unit with recent onset of increasing angina and two hours of severe protracted chest pain. What is the interpretation of this electrocardiogram?

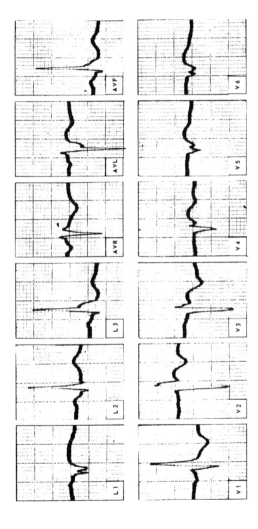

CASE STUDY 70: ANSWER

The rhythm is regular sinus rhythm. The PR interval is normal at .16 sec. QRS duration is .12 sec. There is right bundle branch block as manifest by a rsR' in V1 and terminal S in lead V6. In addition, there is marked right axis deviation with a qR in lead 2, 3 and AVF and a predominantly negative QRS deflection in leads 1 and AVL. This marked right axis in the presence of right bundle branch block suggests posterior hemiblock. In leads V3 to V6, a deep Q wave is present with S-T elevated; T is inverted in V1 to V4. The abnormalities are those of old inferior wall damage and probable recent anteroseptal and lateral wall damage. The presence of right bundle branch block and right axis deviation with a recent anterior wall infarction is often the premonitory of complete heart block and many physicians urge prophylactic temporary cardiac pacemakers be inserted in this situation. Serial tracings should be obtained.

CASE STUDY 71: QUESTION

What is the rhythm? (Lead 2)

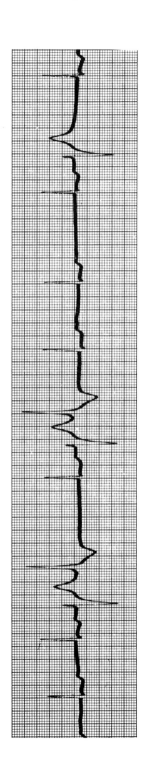

CASE STUDY 71: ANSWER

No P waves are visible. The R-R intervals are totally irregular. The rhythm is atrial fibrillation. Beats #3, 6 and 11 are aberrant and occur at a fixed interval after the preceding R waves. They are coupled ventricular premature contractions (VPCs). Beats #4 and 7 follow the coupled VPCs by varying intervals. These beats have a different QRS configuration. They are either VPCs from a second focus, or, more likely, the VPCs cause aberrant conduction of the following supraventricular QRS complexes. Coupled VPCs in the presence of atrial fibrillation often is a result of digitalis excess. If the patient is receiving digitalis it should be discontinued.

NOTES

What is the diagnosis? The patient was a 30 year-old woman who developed pleuritic chest pain immediately post-partum.

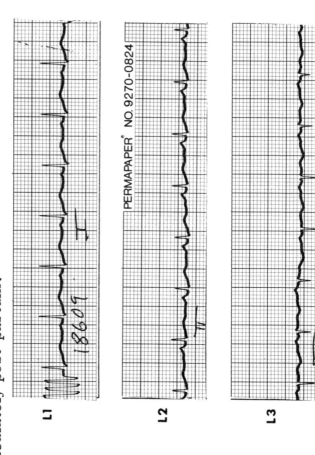

L1

L2

PERMAPAPER® NO. 9270-0824

L3

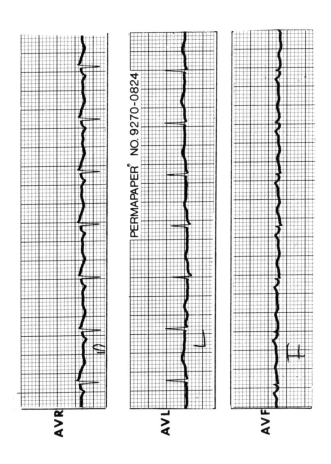

AVR

AVL

AVF

PERMAPAPER® NO. 9270-0824

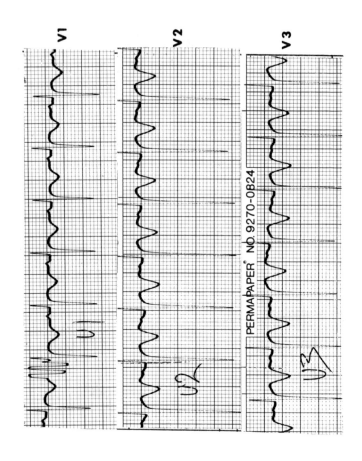

V1

V2

V3

PERMAPAPER® NO. 9270-0824

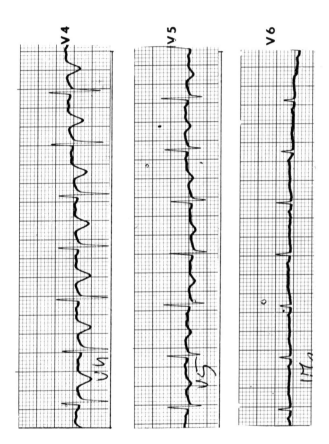

CASE STUDY 72: ANSWER

The rhythm is sinus tachycardia at a rate of 115 beats/min. The significant abnormalities were in precordial leads V_1 to V_5 which showed symmetrically inverted T waves. In addition, there was clockwise rotation of the heart with small r waves in V_1 to V_4. These findings are strongly suggestive of acute cor pulmonale and in this patient pulmonary emboli were documented by lung scan. Normal young individuals may have T wave inversions in the precordial leads but rarely to V_5 and uncommonly to V_4. Serial changes in these T waves would help to confirm the electrocardiographic diagnosis.

CASE STUDY 73: QUESTION

What is the rhythm? Lead 2.

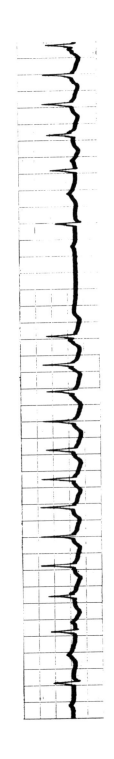

CASE STUDY 73: ANSWER

The first P wave is conducted with a prolonged P-R interval of 0.28 sec. The second P wave appears premature and is followed by a QRS after 0.28 sec. The next P wave is more premature with a prolonged P-R interval of 0.32 sec. The next P wave follows immediately after the third QRS and also has a prolonged P-R interval. The ventricular rate becomes rapid and regular at 185/min. The P waves are superimposed on various portions of the preceding QRS. After this run of tachycardia there is a long pause followed by a P wave with a prolonged P-R interval. The process is then repeated.

The onset of this tachycardia with a premature P wave and a prolonged P-R interval is characteristic of paroxysmal atrial tachycardia. The prolonged pause following the offset is also typical.

NOTES

The tracings shown were obtained at four month intervals. The patient was a 69 year-old man. The first tracing was a routine record during an outpatient visit. The second tracing was obtained on a routine follow-up visit. What is the interpretation of the two tracings and what therapy would be advised?

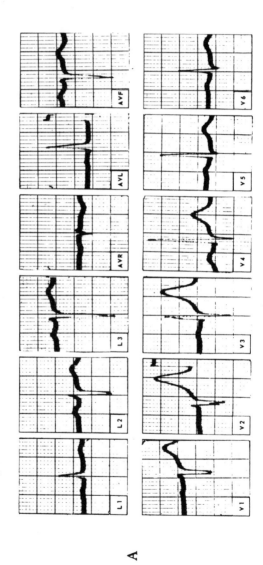

A

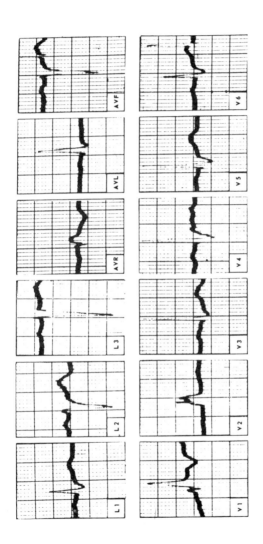

B

Tracing A shows regular sinus rhythm with marked left axis deviation of approximately -60° in the frontal plane. The T waves are tall in V2 and V3. This finding can be seen in normal individuals, but may indicate posterior wall ischemia. In AVL, a standardization artifact masks the T wave. The follow-up tracing B shows that the QRS duration has widened to .14 sec. and right bundle branch block has developed. This is manifest by the rsR' pattern in V1 and V2 and the terminal S wave in leads 1, AVL, V4 to V6. In addition, V1 shows S-T elevation and T inversion which may be due to acute ischemia or may be an artifact secondary to moving baseline. The development of right bundle branch block with pre-existing left axis deviation, (left anterior hemiblock) indicates that the patient now has bifascicular block.

CASE STUDY 75: QUESTION

What is the diagnosis? The patient was a 54 year-old woman with longstanding heart murmurs admitted for increasing congestive failure.

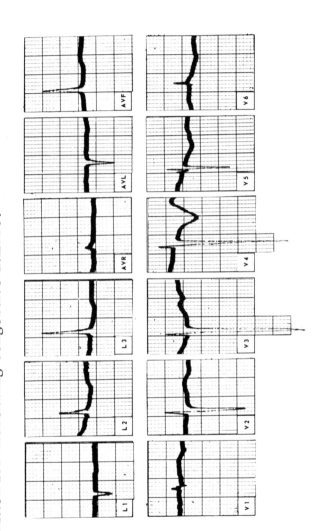

CASE STUDY 75:   ANSWER

The frontal plane electrical axis is markedly rightward beyond $+120^\circ$. There is a dominant R wave in V_1 and clockwise rotation of the heart as manifest by poor r wave progression to V_5 with a deep S wave in V_2 to V_5. These findings are secondary to right
ventricular enlargement. The deep S wave in V_2 to V_4, and RV_6, occurring in a patient
with right ventricular enlargement suggests left ventricular hypertrophy as well. There
are nonspecific S-T abnormalities probably secondary to digitalis effects and myocardial
disease. The rhythm, unclear from this tracing, was atrial fibrillation.

CASE STUDY 76: QUESTION

What is the interpretation of this electrocardiogram obtained on admission to the hospital? The patient is a 73 year-old woman.

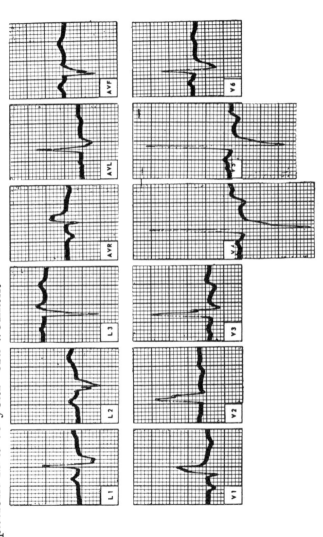

CASE STUDY 76: ANSWER

The rhythm is regular sinus. The QRS duration is .14 second. There is right bundle branch block as manifest by the slurred terminal S waves in leads 1, AVL and V_6, and a slurred terminal R wave in AVR and V_1. There is left axis deviation measuring beyond -45°. There are S-T abnormalities in the precordial leads with T inverted in V_{2-5}. The voltage is somewhat high in V_{4-5}. A qR pattern is present in V_1.

The interpretation is right bundle branch block with abnormal left axis deviation (left anterior hemiblock). The findings indicate bifascicular block involving both the right bundle and the superior ramus of the left bundle. High voltage is not diagnostic of left ventricular hypertrophy when right bundle branch block is present. The S-T abnormalities are non-specific, but suggest myocardial disease or left ventricular hypertrophy. The q in V_1 may be evidence of old anteroseptal infarction. However, this cannot be diagnosed unequivocally as the initial portion of the QRS may be isoelectric.

CASE STUDY 77: QUESTION

Monitor lead. What is the rhythm? The patient has rheumatic heart disease and has been receiving digitalis.

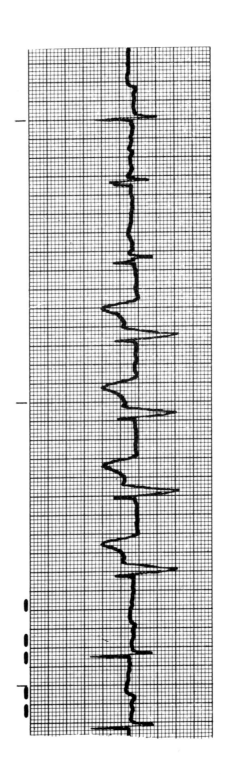

CASE STUDY 77: ANSWER

There are no visible P waves, but atrial fibrillatory waves can be seen. Beats #1 and 2 have a narrow QRS. The following four beats have a wide QRS and are perfectly regular at a rate of 70 beats/min. Beats #7 and 8 are fusion beats intermediate in form between the first two beats and the ensuing four. The last beat is similar to the first two. This regular rhythm interrupting atrial fibrillation represents a parasystolic focus arising below the bifurcation of the Bundle of His. This arrhythmia has been termed either accelerated idioventricular rhythm or a slow ventricular tachycardia. In a patient receiving digitalis, this rhythm usually indicates digitalis toxicity.

NOTES

CASE STUDY 78: QUESTION

What is the diagnosis? Tracing A was a routine record obtained from a 68 year-old woman. The second tracing (B) was obtained following hospitalization for acute pleuritic chest pain.

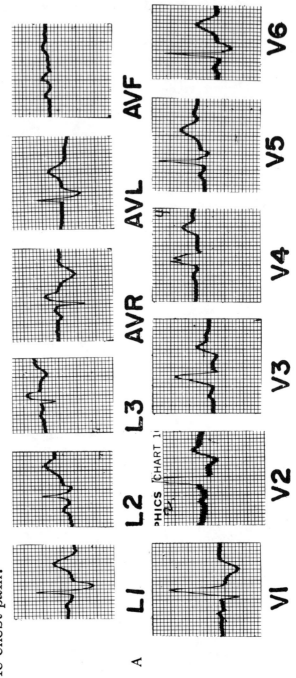

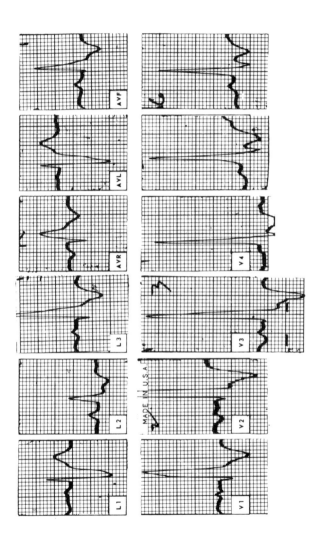

B

CASE STUDY 78: ANSWER

Tracing A shows regular sinus rhythm with a QRS widened to 0.16 sec. The terminal S wave in lead 1, AVL, V_5 and V_6 and terminal R wave in AVR and V_1 are classic manifestations of right bundle branch block. The second tracing shows a marked change in frontal plane mean electrical axis. It is now strikingly rightward with a significantly smaller R wave in lead 1 and tall R wave in lead 3 and AVF. In addition, T is deeply inverted in V_3 to V_6. The development of marked right axis deviation in the presence of right bundle branch block suggests posterior hemiblock. However, in this patient, the abnormality appeared during the course of multiple acute pulmonary emboli. It, therefore, appeared more likely that it was secondary to acute cor pulmonale rather than posterior hemiblock. The P wave in lead 2 is somewhat peaked suggesting P pulmonale but is not diagnostic. The T wave changes in the precordial leads are nonspecific and could be due to ischemia.

NOTES

CASE STUDY 79: QUESTION

ECG obtained from a 14 year-old black male. What is the interpretation?

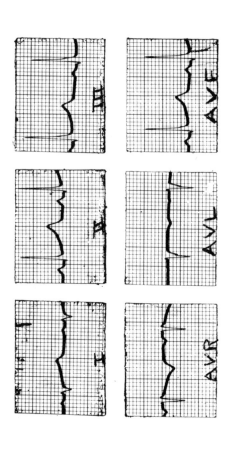

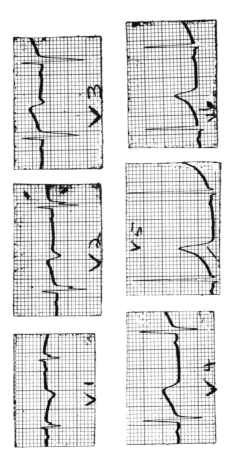

CASE STUDY 79: ANSWER

The rhythm is sinus. The mean electrical axis is approximately 100° in the frontal plane. There are terminal T wave inversions in V_2 and V_3. The S-T segment is elevated in lead 2 and V_{4-6}. The elevation is primarily due to elevation of the J point.

These S-T and T wave changes are a normal variant in young individuals.

NOTES

CASE STUDY 80: QUESTION

What is the rhythm? Continuous Lead 2.

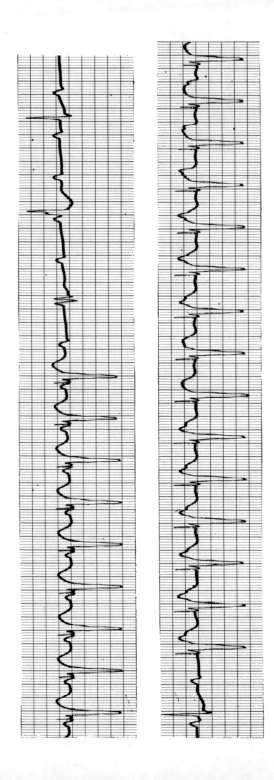

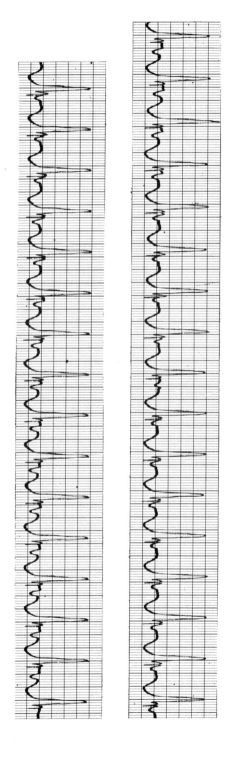

CASE STUDY 80: ANSWER

The initial nine beats show a pacemaker spike preceding each QRS with a fixed PR interval. Following the ninth QRS the pacemaker was turned off. The ensuing P wave is non-conducted and the QRS following it is a ventricular escape beat. The next three escape beats arise, in all likelihood, from the AV junction as the QRS is relatively narrow. The pacemaker function resumes after the first escape beat in strip two and evidence of atrial activity can be seen buried on the T waves.

The tracing demonstrates that in the absence of the pacemaker, there is complete heart block and junctional or ventricular escape beats. The bottom two strips show the P wave remaining in close proximity to the ventricular paced beats. This phenomenon is known as synchronization, and could be demonstrated repeatedly by turning the pacemaker off and on. When the pacer was turned to a more rapid or slower rate, the P waves were no longer temporally related to the ventricular complex.

CASE STUDY 81: QUESTION

The patient is a 71 year-old man who fainted and was brought to the Emergency Room. What is the diagnosis?

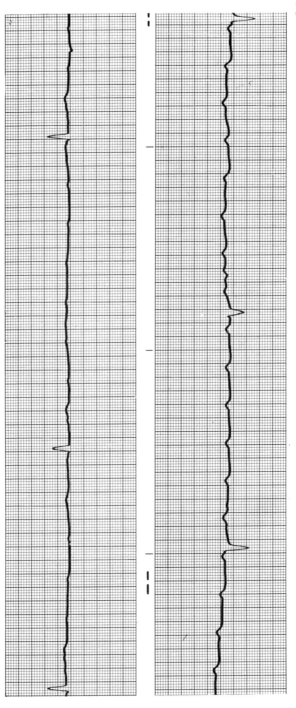

CASE STUDY 81: ANSWER

The atrial rate is 110 and regular. The QRS is .12 sec. The ventricular rate is approx-imately 18 beats/minute and is slightly irregular. The patient has complete heart block and a very slow idioventricular pacemaker. A cardiac pacemaker should be inserted.

CASE STUDY 82: QUESTION

This tracing was obtained four days following cardiac surgery to repair a stenotic mitral valve. What is the interpretation?

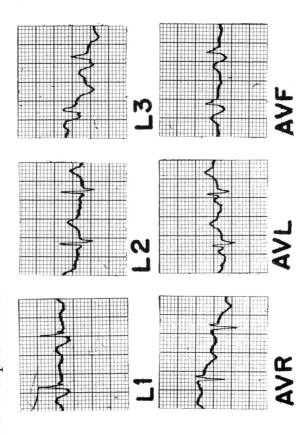

CASE STUDY 82: ANSWER

The rhythm is regular sinus rhythm. The tracing shows a depressed PR segment in leads 1, 3, AVF, and elevation of the PR segment in AVR. S-T is elevated in leads 1, 3, and AVF. The PR segment abnormalities have been reported to occur when there is atrial pericarditis, although other forms of atrial pathology can produce such changes. The S-T elevations are consistent with classic pericarditis and are not uncommonly seen in the immediate post-operative period following heart surgery.

CASE STUDY 83: QUESTION

Lead 2 taken during carotid sinus massage. What is the interpretation?

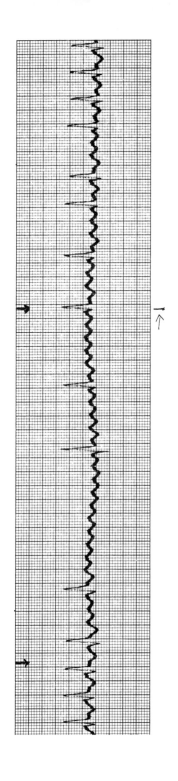

CASE STUDY 83: ANSWER

The first four QRS complexes are almost regular at a rate of 150/min. With carotid massage, there is marked slowing of the ventricular rate. Distinct flutter waves can be seen. Following cessation of massage the ventricular rate speeds up to a rate of 150/min. for the last four beats.

This response to carotid massage is characteristic of flutter with transient slowing of the ventricular rate. The diagnosis of atrial flutter can readily be made from the clear demonstration of flutter waves during ventricular slowing. In this patient, the diagnosis of flutter was not apparent when the rate was rapid.

NOTES

What is the diagnosis? The patient was a 60 year-old man admitted to the hospital with severe congestive failure. Tracing A was obtained on admission. Tracing B was obtained one week later when his failure improved.

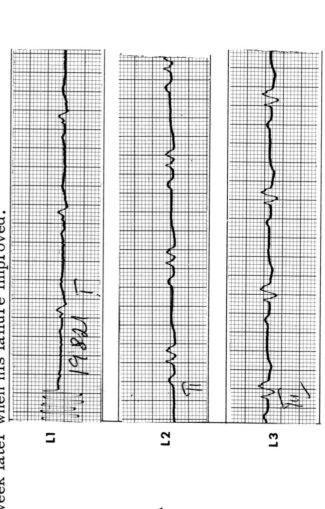

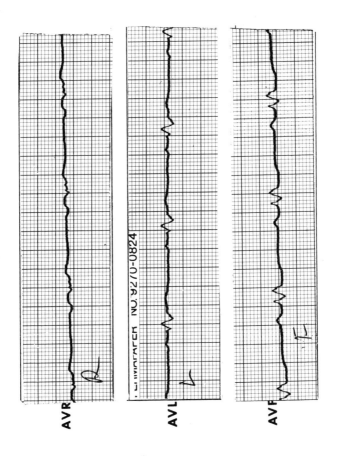

AVR

AVL

AVF

NO. 92/0-0824

A
(cont'd)

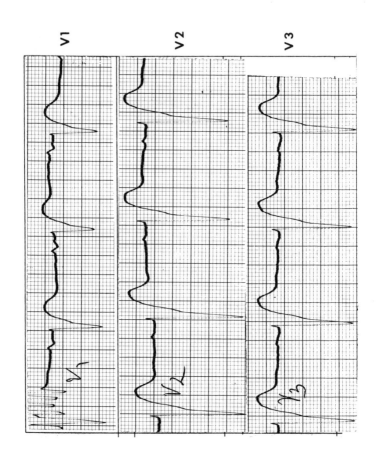

A
(cont'd)

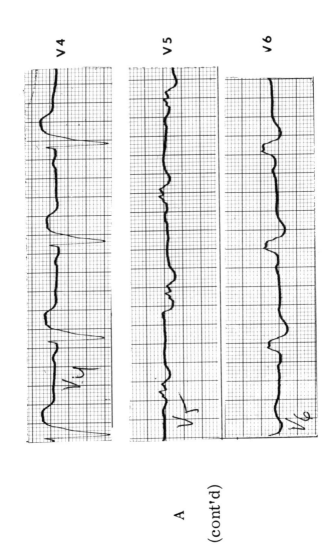

V4

V5

V6

A
(cont'd)

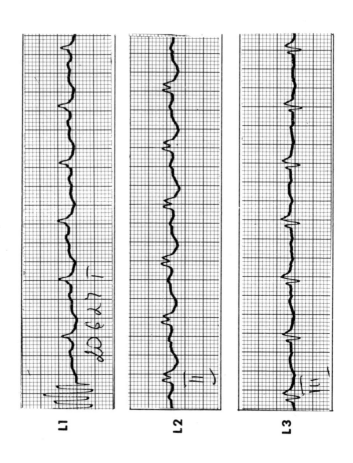

L1

L2

L3

B

221

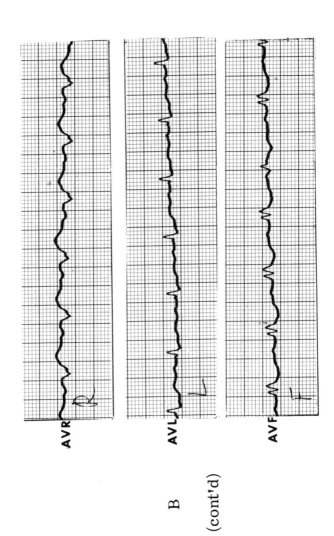

B

(cont'd)

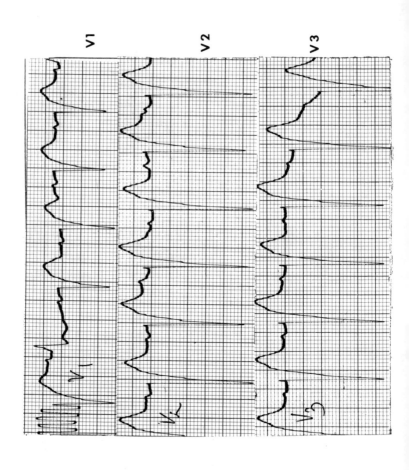

B

(cont'd)

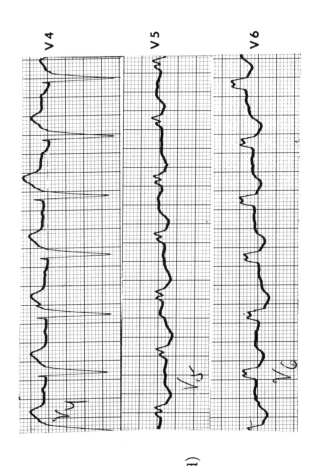

B
(cont'd)

223

CASE STUDY 84: ANSWER

In tracing A the rhythm is regular sinus rhythm with a rate of 57 beats/minute. The PR interval is 0.20 sec. The QRS duration is 0.21 sec. The configuration is that of left bundle branch block with no visible septal Q wave in lead 1 or V_6. This marked widening of the QRS is an unusual prolongation, as left bundle branch block characteristically has a QRS duration of 0.12–.14 sec. The patient's follow-up tracing (B) shows left bundle branch block with a QRS duration of only 0.13 sec. The improved ventricular conduction suggests better myocardial oxygenation. The first beat in V_1 (tracing B) is either a late ventricular extrasystole or a conducted beat showing right bundle branch block.

CASE STUDY 85: QUESTION

The patient is a 53 year-old man with a history of hospitalization several years previously following a bout of chest pain. What is the interpretation of this electrocardiogram?

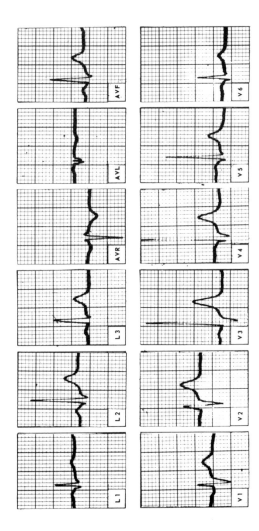

CASE STUDY 85: ANSWER

The rhythm is regular sinus. The sole abnormality appears in lead AVL where there is a Q wave and inverted T wave with upright P wave. This is strongly suggestive of old lateral or apical myocardial infarction ... and upon reviewing this patient's hospital records, this was found to have been the diagnosis.

NOTES

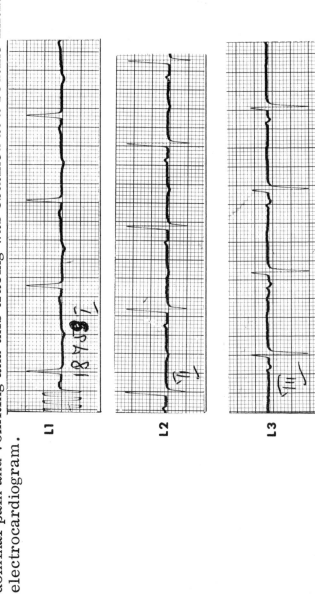

CASE STUDY 86: QUESTION

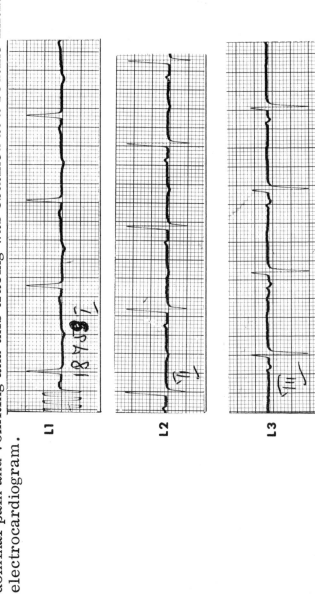

What is the diagnosis? The patient was a 70 year-old woman admitted with severe abdominal pain and vomiting and this tracing was obtained at a routine initial admission electrocardiogram.

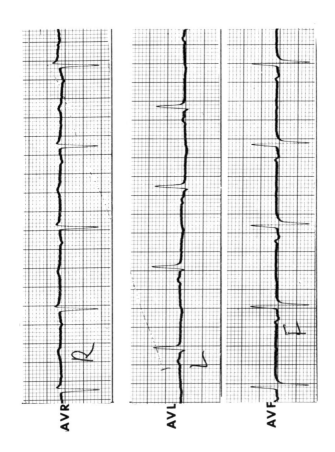

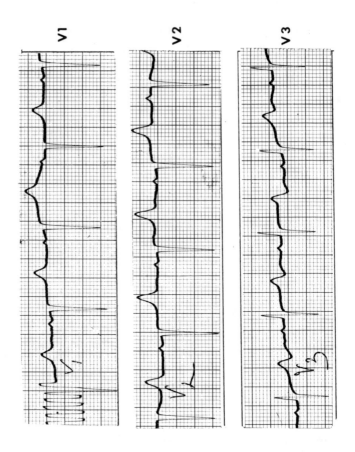

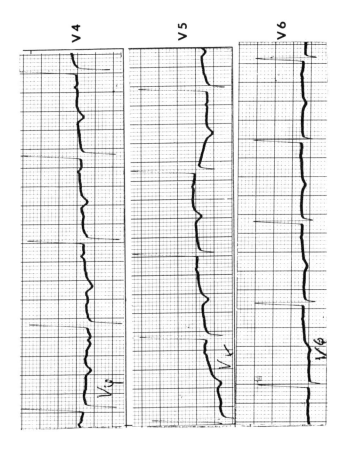

CASE STUDY 86: ANSWER

The rhythm is regular sinus with a PR interval of 0.16 sec. and a QRS duration of 0.09. The heart rate is 69 beats per minute. The Q-T interval is prolonged to 0.48 sec. This long QT interval is primarily due to prolongation of the S-T segment as the T wave is relatively narrow. T is inverted in leads 1, 2, AVL, V_4 to V_6. The prolonged QT interval with a relatively narrow T wave is strongly suggestive of hypocalcemia. This patient had acute pancreatitis with a low serum calcium level. The T wave abnormalities were secondary to coronary artery disease.

CASE STUDY 87: QUESTION

Lead 2. What is the rhythm? Patient has cor pulmonale of long standing and has been receiving digoxin for congestive heart failure and a rapid heart rate.

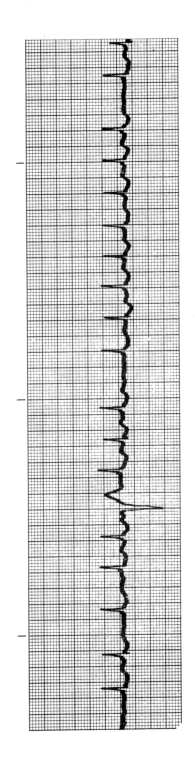

CASE STUDY 87: ANSWER

No P waves are visible. The undulations between the R waves are the f waves of atrial fibrillation. Beat #6 is aberrantly conducted and represents a ventricular premature contraction. Beats 11 to 14 are almost precisely regular as are beats 15 to 17. The regularization of the ventricular response in patients with atrial fibrillation suggests digitalis toxicity. When it occurs at a very rapid rate, it probably represents a junctional tachycardia. It is impossible at times to determine from the electrocardiogram whether or not digitalis should be discontinued or increased. It is usually safer to stop the drug and observe the patient's response. Digoxin levels may be of help.

CASE STUDY 88: QUESTION

What is the diagnosis? The patient was a 42 year-old woman admitted to the hospital with pressing anterior chest pain of four hours duration.

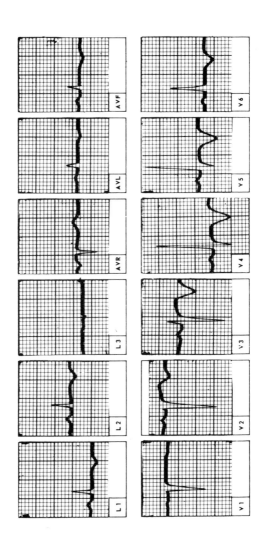

CASE STUDY 88: ANSWER

This tracing shows symmetrically inverted T waves in leads 1, 2, AVL, AVF, V_2 to V_6. The S-T segment is slightly elevated in V_2 and V_3. These abnormalities suggest antero-lateral ischemia or infarction of indeterminate age. The suspicion of recent damage was high in view of the S-T elevations and the symmetrically inverted deep T waves. This patient was of interest as there was no evidence of acute myocardial infarction on serial blood studies. Coronary angiograms performed shortly thereafter showed normal coro-nary arteries, with an akinetic area in the left ventricle. The syndrome of myocardial infarction, or S-T-T abnormalities in relatively young women with normal coronary ar-teries is as yet inadequately explained. The electrocardiographic abnormalities, such as demonstrated by this patient, can be striking.

CASE STUDY 89: QUESTION

What is the rhythm? Electrocardiogram obtained during the initial stages of an acute myocardial infarction. Lead II.

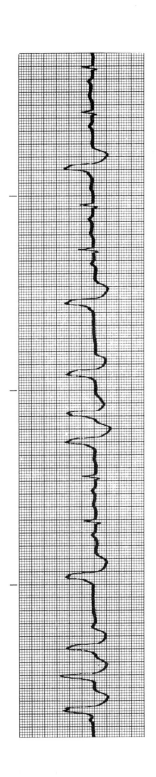

CASE STUDY 89: ANSWER

The rhythm is regular sinus rhythm with a rate of 85 beats/min. The sinus rhythm is interrupted frequently by bursts of irregular ventricular premature beats. Sinus rhythm is uninterrupted as can be determined by plotting the P-P intervals which are regular. The rhythm may be termed a chaotic ventricular arrhythmia or ventricular tachycardia. Its gross irregularity is unusual. Anti-arrhythmic therapy is indicated.

NOTES

CASE STUDY 90: QUESTION

The patient was an 81 year-old man admitted to the hospital in acute pulmonary edema. The V leads are half-standardized. What is the diagnosis and what is the arrhythmia?

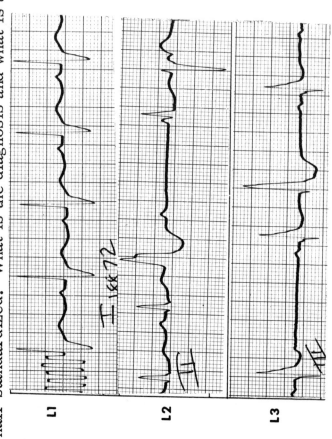

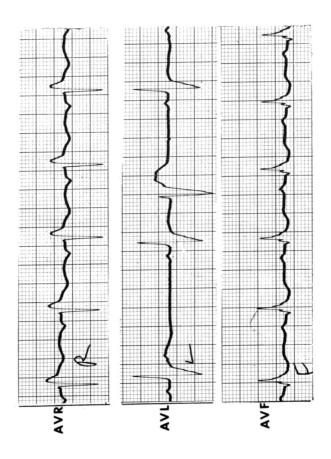

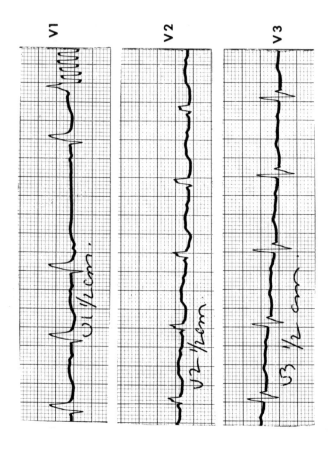

V1

V2

V3

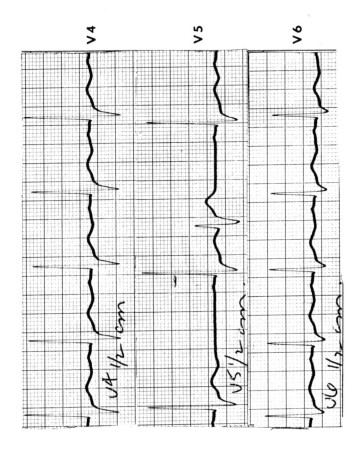

V4

V5

V6

CASE STUDY 90: ANSWER

The rhythm is regular sinus rhythm with a PR interval of 0.16 sec. and QRS duration of 0.14 sec. In lead 2, there is a ventricular premature contraction followed by a nonconducted P wave. This indicates that the ventricular premature contraction penetrated the AV junction in a retrograde fashion making the AV node refractory. This is an example of concealed retrograde conduction. Following the nonconducted P wave, there is a junctional escape beat with a P wave superimposed. A premature aberrant beat follows the junctional escape beat. This premature aberrant beat probably arises in the His-Purkinje system and at a higher level than the VPC, as it is followed by a negative P wave proving retrograde conduction has occurred. In lead 3, AVL, V_1 and V_5, there are long pauses. The S-T segment of the beat prior to the pause is deformed by a premature P wave. This is a nonconducted atrial premature contraction. Following the long R-R interval, there is a short R-R with a QRS configuration that is aberrant, but not markedly so. The latter beats are, in all likelihood, junctional in origin with aberration. The contour of the normally conducted QRS complexes is that of right bundle branch block. The small Q waves in 3 and AVF may indicate old inferior wall infarction.

NOTES

CASE STUDY 91: QUESTION

246

What is the diagnosis? The patient was a 49 year-old woman admitted to the hospital hypotensive, with complaints of anterior chest pain of several hours duration.

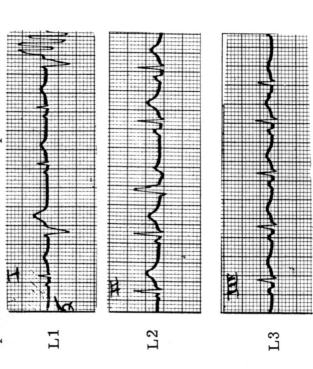

L1

L2

L3

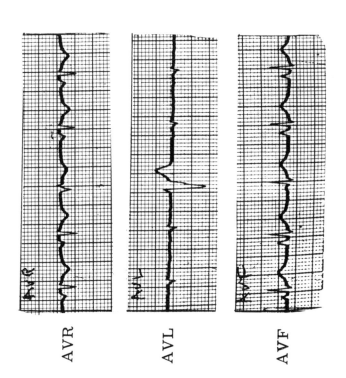

AVR

AVL

AVF

247

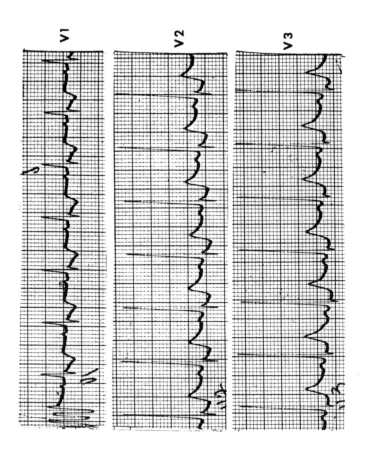

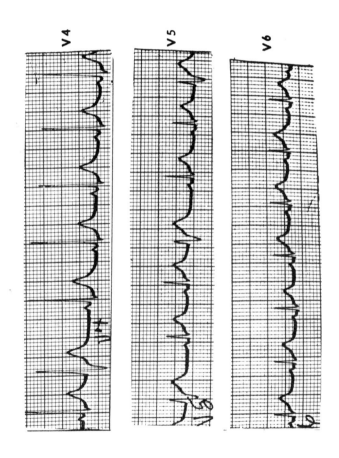

CASE STUDY 91: ANSWER

The rhythm is sinus tachycardia with a rate of 100 beats/min. There are ventricular premature contractions visible in leads 1, 2, AVL, V_4 and V_5. There is an atrial premature contraction in lead 3, and in AVF a wandering atrial pacemaker causes variation in the P wave configuration. Lead V_1 shows a tall R wave significantly taller than the S. There are S–T depressions in leads V_1 to V_3. The standard leads show no abnormalities. The findings in leads V_1 to V_3 could indicate posterolateral myocardial infarction. The possibility of acute right ventricular enlargement secondary to pulmonary emboli might be considered, but the absence of P pulmonale or right axis deviation would be somewhat against this diagnosis. This patient died several hours following this electrocardiogram and post–mortem examination revealed rupture of the heart secondary to posterolateral myocardial infarction. Her electrocardiogram obtained a year prior to this tracing had been completely normal.

CASE STUDY 92: QUESTION

What is the rhythm? (Lead 2)

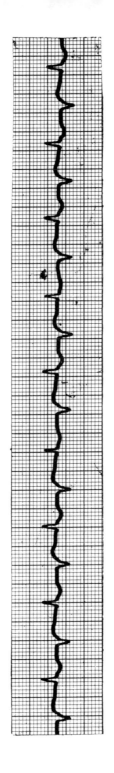

CASE STUDY 92: ANSWER

The ventricular rate is 150. No atrial activity is visible. Every alternate QRS is aberrantly conducted, but each has a QRS duration which is narrow at less than 0.11 sec. This is a bidirectional tachycardia. Since the QRS duration is narrow, the beats are supraventricular in origin arising above the bifurcation of the bundle of His. Each alternate beat takes a different pathway producing the variation in conduction. In a patient on digitalis, such an arrhythmia is indicative of digitalis toxicity.

CASE STUDY 93: QUESTION

What is the rhythm? Lead 2.

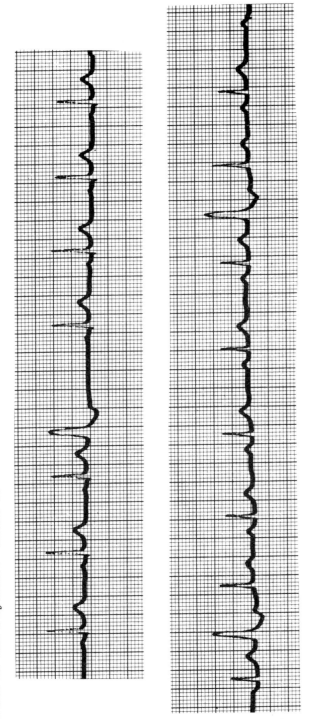

CASE STUDY 93: ANSWER

The rhythm is sinus rhythm at the rate of 75 beats/min. The fourth beat is a ventricular premature contraction with a fully compensatory pause. The second strip shows two VPCs which are interpolated. These are followed by P-R prolongation. This P-R prolongation following an interpolated VPC indicates that there is concealed retrograde conduction from the ventricular premature contraction into A-V junctional tissue.

CASE STUDY 94: QUESTION

67 year-old man with congestive failure. What is the interpretation of this ECG?

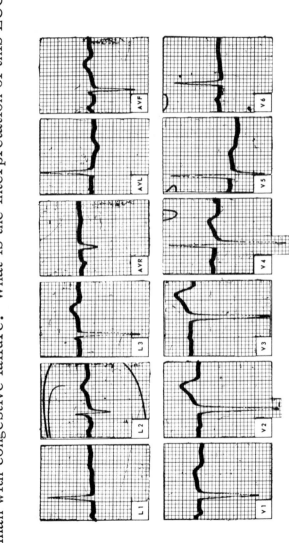

CASE STUDY 94: ANSWER

The rhythm is regular sinus rhythm. There is left axis deviation with a mean electrical axis of greater than -30°. The R in AVL measures 13 mm. The S V2 + R V5 measures 37 mm. ST is depressed in 1 and AVL with T biphasic. There is a QS pattern in V1-3 with positive T waves. These abnormalities represent myocardial disease with probable left ventricular hypertrophy. The abnormal left axis deviation suggests conduction block in the superior branch of the left bundle (left anterior hemiblock). The QS pattern in V1-3 may represent an anteroseptal infarction, but this pattern may be seen without in-farction, especially when there is marked left axis deviation.

NOTES

CASE STUDY 95: QUESTION

What is the diagnosis? The patient was admitted with documented bony metastases.

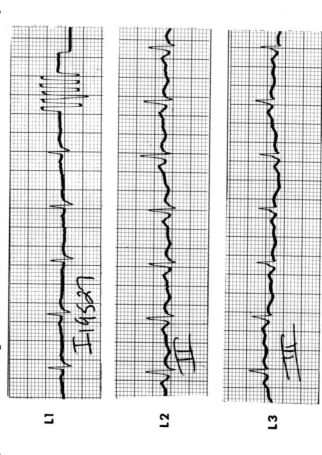

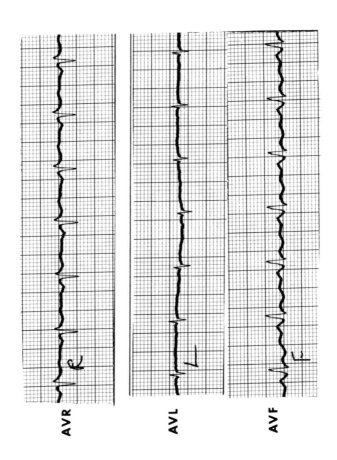

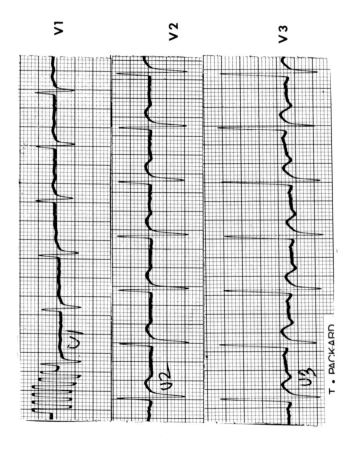

T . PACKARD

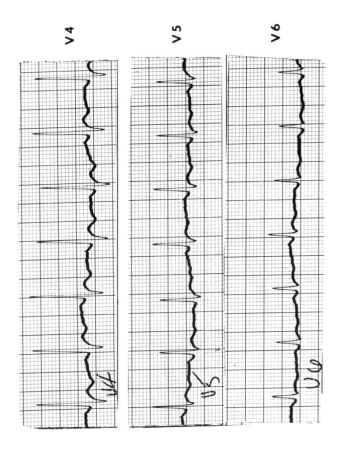

V4

V5

V6

CASE STUDY 95: ANSWER

The rhythm is sinus tachycardia with a rate of 110 beats/min. The QT interval is 0.27 sec. There are nonspecific T wave abnormalities in 1, 2, 3, AVF, V_3 to V_6. The relatively short QT was suspicious of hypercalcemia in a patient not receiving digitalis. Serum calcium determinations were elevated to 13 to 14 mg.%.

CASE STUDY 96: QUESTION

What is the rhythm? (Lead V1)

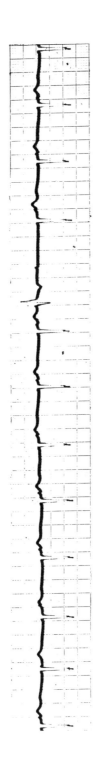

CASE STUDY 96: ANSWER

The ventricular rate is approximately 75 per minute, but is slightly irregular. Note that the P wave is buried in the ST segment. It is upright and occurs at varying distances from the preceding QRS. Possibly it is a retrograde P wave. An alternate explanation is that the P wave is antegrade and conducts to the succeeding QRS, with a P-R interval of .68 sec. Proof that the latter is indeed the case is obtained by observing beat #2, in which there is no P wave in the S-T segment, but the P wave is superimposed on the terminal portion of the QRS. If one measures this P-R interval, it is precisely the same as the usual P-R interval. Note that the R-R interval encompassing this P wave is appropriately shortened. Secondly, following the VPC seen after beat #8, the P wave is now clearly visible, is obviously not retrograde, and has precisely the same P-R interval as the previous P-R intervals. The interpretation, therefore, is regular sinus rhythm, first degree heart block with a P-R interval of .68 second, occasional ventricular premature contractions. The P wave following beat #8 is not conducted because it is blocked by the ventricular premature contraction.

CASE STUDY 97: QUESTION

What is the interpretation? Long lead 2.

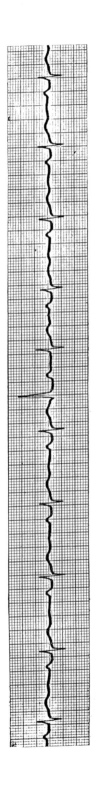

CASE STUDY 97: ANSWER

The rhythm is regular sinus rhythm with 1° A-V block. The P-R interval is .24 second. Following beat #5, there is a ventricular premature contraction which is interpolated. The ensuing P-R interval is prolonged to .36 second. This prolongation indicates concealed retrograde conduction into the A-V junction delaying the conduction of the ensuing P wave.

CASE STUDY 98: QUESTION

What is the rhythm? Strip A is lead 2. Strip B an intra-atrial lead.

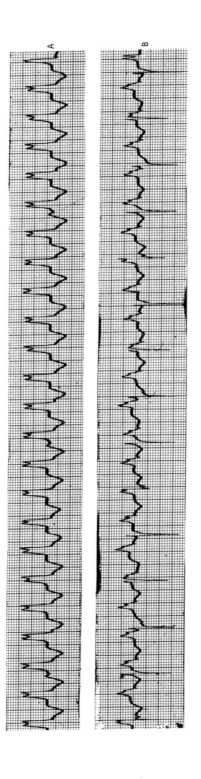

CASE STUDY 98: ANSWER

The QRS complexes are 0.14 second in duration. The ventricular rate is regular at a rate of 138/min. Atrial activity can be seen in lead 2 preceding the third QRS and in the S-T segment of the fourth. The intra-atrial lead clearly demonstrates these P waves at least ten times larger than in lead 2. Intra-atrial leads are very helpful in identifying atrial activity in tachycardias especially with aberrant ventricular conduction.

The atrial rate is 85/min; the ventricular rate is 137/min. Both are regular. The tachycardia is ventricular in origin.

NOTES

CASE STUDY 99: QUESTION

Tracings obtained at 2 hour intervals. What is the interpretation?

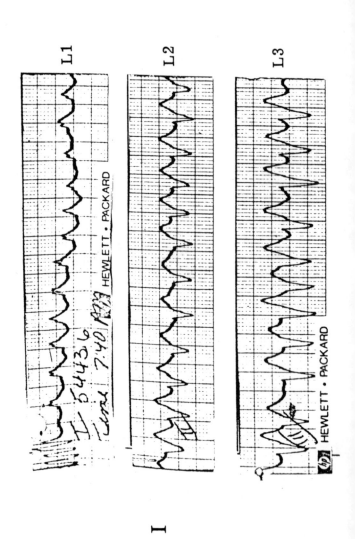

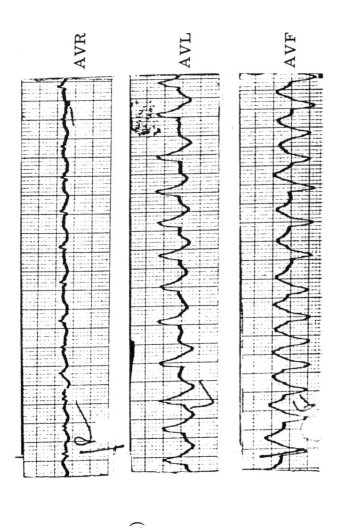

I
(cont'd)

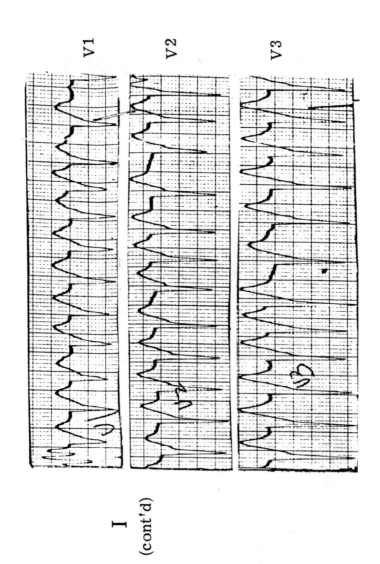

V1

V2

V3

I
(cont'd)

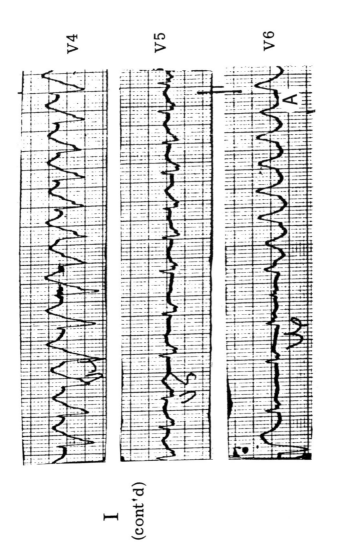

V4

V5

V6

A

I
(cont'd)

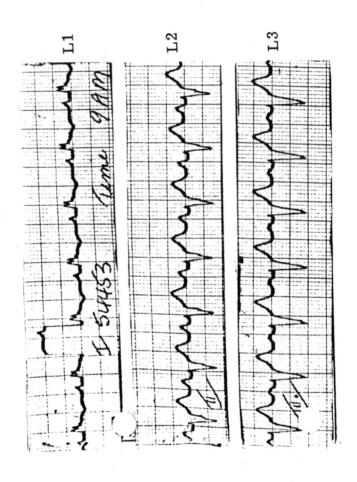

L1

L2

L3

I 54453   Time 9 A.M

II

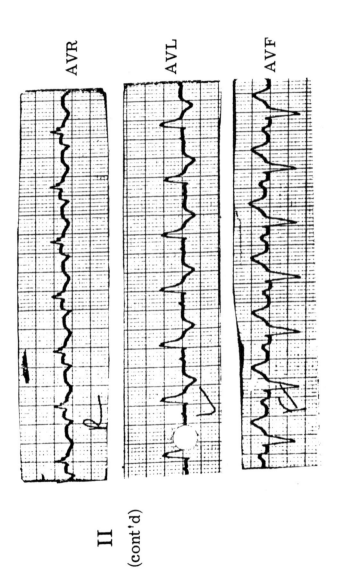

AVR

AVL

AVF

II
(cont'd)

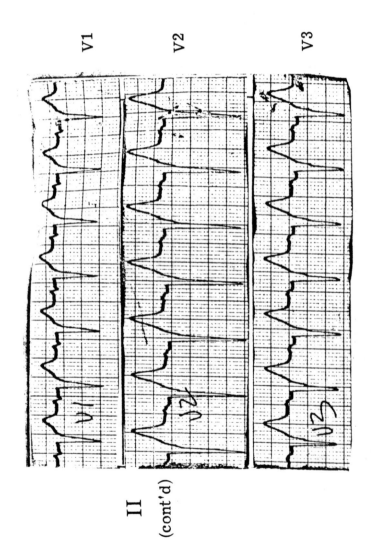

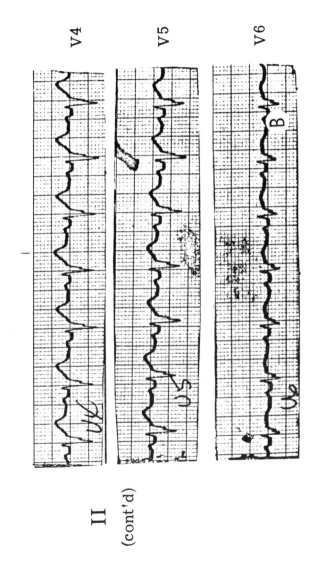

V4

V5

V6

II
(cont'd)

CASE STUDY 99: ANSWER

In the first tracing, the QRS is aberrantly conducted and widened. There is marked left axis deviation. Note that the QRS varies in duration. This is especially visible in V6, where the more rapid ventricular complexes are more aberrant. The rhythm in the first record is atrial fibrillation with aberrant ventricular conduction of the left bundle branch block variety. The last beats in lead V6 resemble ventricular tachycardia, but the gross irregularity makes this diagnosis less likely.

In the second tracing, the rhythm is sinus rhythm with notched P waves and biphasic P waves in V1. The QRS is .11 seconds with Q waves in 1 and AVL. The mean electrical axis in the frontal plane is still minus 60°; clockwise rotation is present in horizontal plane. The patient has an intraventricular conduction delay with block of the superior ramus of the left bundle (left anterior hemiblock). When the rate accelerates, as in tracing 1, left bundle branch block occurs, with persistent LAD.

CASE STUDY 100: QUESTION

What is the rhythm? Lead 2.

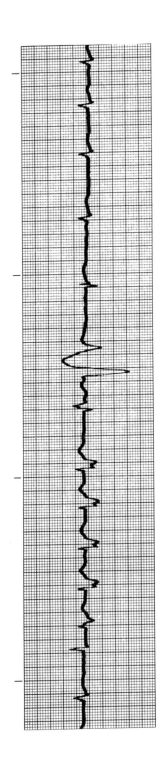

CASE STUDY 100: ANSWER

The rhythm is irregular and no P waves are seen; f waves are visible. The underlying rhythm is atrial fibrillation. Beats #3 to 7 are aberrantly conducted, are precisely regular and at a rate of approximately 110 beats/min. Beat #9 is a ventricular premature contraction. The ensuing beats are irregular. Beats #3 to 7 represent accelerated idioventricular rhythm. In a patient receiving digitalis, this would represent digitalis toxicity.

A

Angina Pectoris, 18
Artifact, 30
Ashman phenomenon, 158
Atrial:
   arrhythmia, 90
     chaotic, 90
   bigeminy, 62
   fibrillation, 158, 178, 196, 234, 278, 280
   flutter, 30, 214
   premature beat, 10, 20, 62, 244, 250
   premature beat blocked, 244
   premature beat with aberrant conduction, 78
   septal defect, 106
   synchronous pacemaker, 60
   tachycardia, 70, 118, 136, 168, 186
     multifocal, 90
A-V:
   dissociation, 66
   junctional escape beats, 244
   junctional rhythm, 66

B

Bilateral bundle branch block, 22
Biventricular hypertrophy, 192
Bradytachyarrhythmia, 118

C

Carotid sinus massage, 214
Combined ventricular hypertrophy, 128, 192
Concealed conduction, 244, 254, 266
Cor pulmonale, acute, 110, 184, 200

D

Delta wave, 8
Dextrocardia, 82
Digitalis toxicity, 70, 136, 178, 234, 252, 280